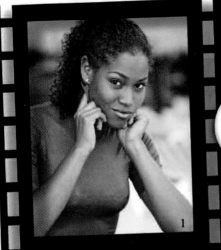
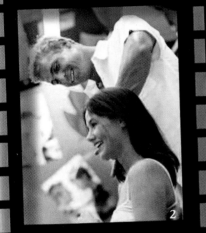
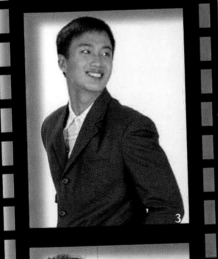
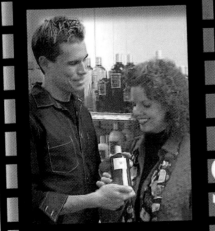

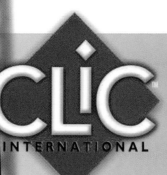

CLiC
INTERNATIONAL

CERTIFIED LEARNING IN COSMETOLOGY®

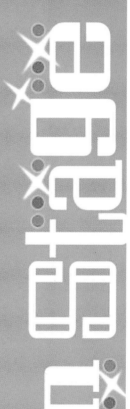

On Stage

success dynamics

INTRODUCTION

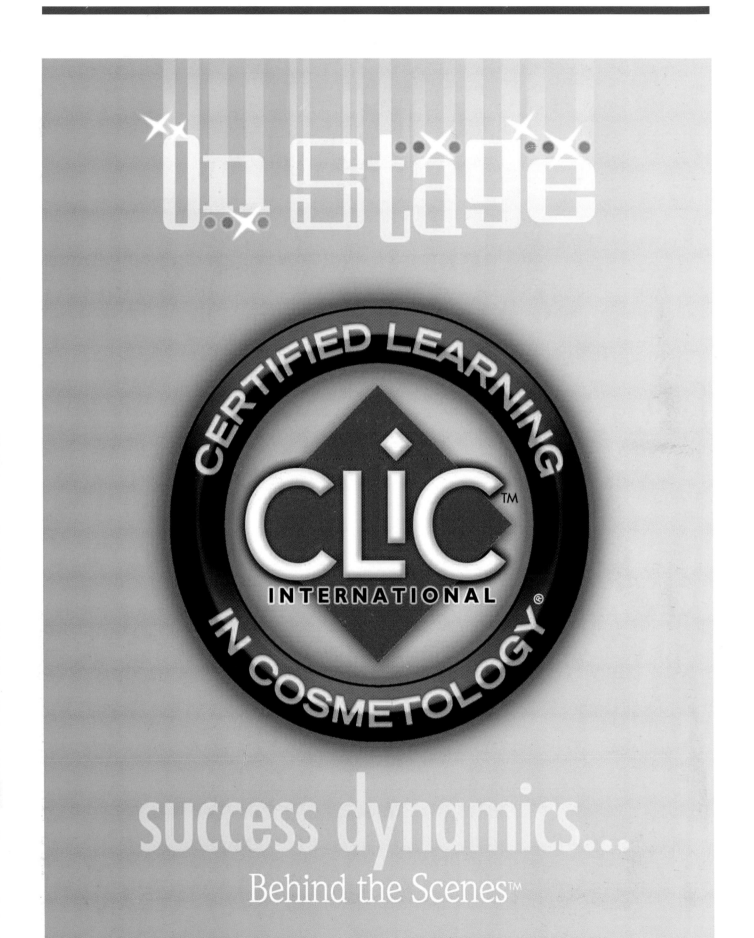

On Stage

CERTIFIED LEARNING
CLiC™
INTERNATIONAL
IN COSMETOLOGY®

success dynamics...
Behind the Scenes™

Welcome to ...

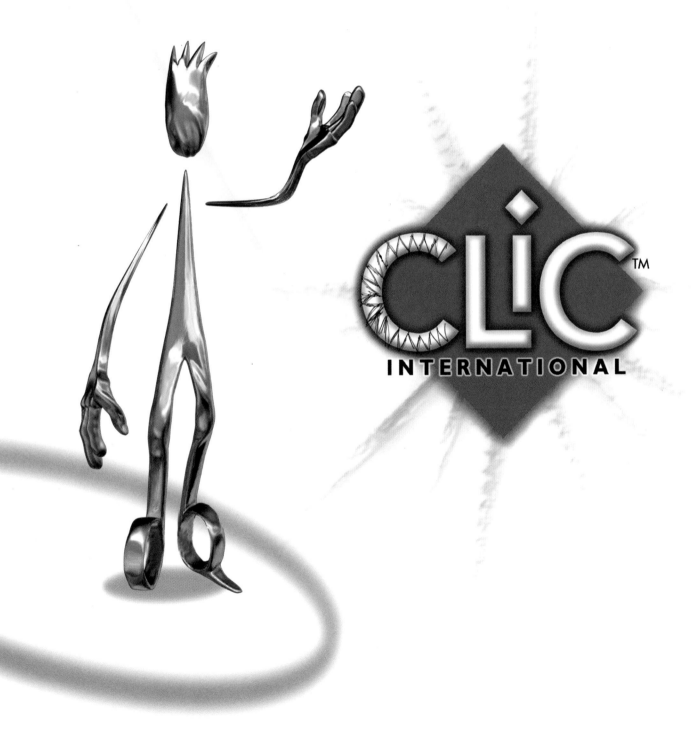

CLiC™
INTERNATIONAL

Dedication ...

To all of the professionals who share the gift of beauty with every individual they touch ... may you find success and personal rewards as you embark upon your career! We applaud you for helping create beauty in the world.

"Make each performance with every client deserve a standing ovation."

From Geno & Shaunna:
We worked with an extraordinary group of creative people, each of whom deserves special thanks. Frank Schoeneman and Randy Rick provided the vision and artistic inspiration. Amanda Condict and her amazing team of graphic artists and photographers including Denise, Barb, Layne, Michelle, Flora, Jessica, Stefan and Bonnie worked tirelessly to ensure that each page was visually exciting. Victoria Sutherland's editorial skills were invaluable. Sallie Bengtson kept everyone on track by coordinating the team's efforts. Kate Troc and Jayne Morehouse reviewed the manuscript and provided valuable feedback.

Additional thanks from Geno:
A special thanks to Sam, Holly, Steve, Terri, Kimberly, John, Maryanne, Tom, Paul, JP, Jack, Phillip, Mario, Peter, Chuck & Deb, Behind the Chair, Hair Color & Design and Bob, TSA especially Jill , The NCA, Intercoiffure, The ICSA, The IHE, Nailpro especially Debra, and my family for their support. Also, thanks for the endless support and friendship from all of the great beauty professionals who take the time to work with me and keep my message alive in the salon where it matters most. They have no idea how small life would be without them.

Additional thanks from Shaunna:
Very special thanks to Jim, Tracy, Claire, Marie, Mary, Theresa, Margie, Cathy, Charlie, Mike, Melanie, Abe, and my family for their support and encouragement.

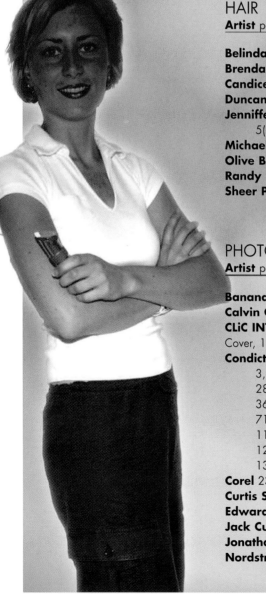

HAIR
Artist page(picture number)

Belinda Baker 153(3)
Brenda Petty 153(4)
Candice Hodges 5(1)
Duncan Lai 153(6, 8)
Jenniffer & Company
 5(2, 3), 153(7)
Michael Rocco 153(1)
Olive Benson 153(5)
Randy Rick 153(2)
Sheer Professionals Salon 10(1)

PHOTOGRAPHY
Artist page(picture number)

Banana Stock 1(2)
Calvin Childs 5(1)
CLiC INTERNATIONAL Art Team
Cover, 11
Condict & Company
 3, 4, 9, 16, 22, 23(2), 24, 26,
 28, 31(2), 32(1), 33, 35(3),
 36, 37, 39(1), 41(2), 50, 53(2),
 71, 80, 88, 92, 99, 100, 102(1),
 110(4), 117, 118, 119, 121, 122,
 123(2), 126, 127, 128, 129(2),
 130(2), 131(2), 147, 151, 154
Corel 23(1), 60(1)
Curtis Spratlin 153(5)
Edward Tytel 153(4)
Jack Cutler 153(1)
Jonathan Martin 153(3)
Nordstrom 111(1)

Photos.Com
 1(1,3), 3, 6, 7, 10, 14(1,2),
 15(2), 16, 20, 25, 29, 32(2),
 35(2), 42, 43, 48, 51, 52, 56,
 57, 58, 59, 60(2), 61, 62, 63,
 64, 68, 69, 70, 75(1), 76, 77,
 78, 79, 81, 82, 86, 87, 89, 90,
 91, 92, 93, 98, 99, 102, 103,
 104, 105, 106, 110(1,2,3),
 111(2), 113, 114, 120), 123(1),
 125, 129(1), 130(1), 131(1),
 132, 146, 147, 148, 149, 150,
 151, 152, 155
Rubberball 7
Tom Carson
 5(2,3), 10(2), 153(2,7)
Victoria Sutherland
 9, 14(3), 15(1), 16, 18, 21, 27,
 30, 31(1), 32(3), 35(1), 38,
 39(2), 40, 41(1,3), 72, 75(2),
 88, 89, 92, 95, 96, 97, 101,
 102(2), 154(2)

"A special thanks to all the professionals who provided their photo images to support the education of future stylists."

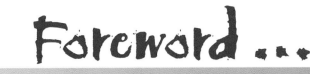

Foreword ...

Sir Isaac Newton once said, "If I have been able to see further, it was only because I stood on the shoulders of giants." This profound statement represents one of the guiding principles of the Certified Learning in Cosmetology™ (CLiC) system. There is much to be learned and discovered by "standing on the shoulders of giants." It is only by studying the discoveries and accomplishments of the leaders who came before us that we can prepare for the future.

The CLiC system provides a broad cosmetology education with a focus on three key areas:

1. A basic cosmetology foundation
2. An introduction to artistic concepts and visual inspiration to nurture creativity
3. Effective interpersonal, sales and retail techniques

Although the cosmetology industry is continually evolving, its basic foundation remains unchanged.
The foundation of cosmetology is an understanding of human biology combined with scientific and mathematic concepts used to create the desired results. Building on the basic foundation of cosmetology, artistic concepts and visual inspiration are used to develop and nurture creativity. Throughout the foundational and artistic learning process, successful interpersonal, selling and retailing skills are introduced and practiced. These skills are paramount to the financial success of the professional cosmetologist.

You will find CLiC to be a visually exciting and inspirational education system focused on preparing students to be salon ready upon completion of their studies. Developed by an industry giant himself, master hair designer and international award winner Randy Rick is the creative force behind this revolutionary CLiC system. Always a step ahead, Mr. Rick developed the CLiC system of learning to elevate the artistic and practical skills of today's students. Through the CLiC program, he shares his vast international knowledge and experience with you, the cosmetology professional of the future!

CLiC to a dynamic future in the world of beauty!

CLiC™
INTERNATIONAL

The CLiC Education Team ...

The CLiC Education Team represents more than 100 years of combined cosmetology industry education, experience and wisdom. The team includes international award winners, top educators, stylists, salon and beauty school owners, operations managers and owner/operators of highly successful cosmetology businesses.

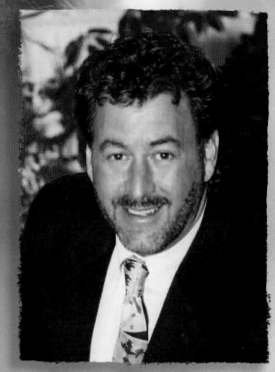

About the Authors

Geno Stampora, a recipient of many beauty industry awards, is a licensed cosmetologist, industry educator and life enhancement speaker. He has owned, managed and operated salons, spas, beauty academies and a professional beauty supply distributorship. His life enhancement seminars are in great demand and he has lectured all over the world. As a consultant, he has worked with the world's finest salons, contributing fundamentals for marketing, communication and people skills.

He works closely with industry trade magazines and has published numerous articles. Geno and his family live in northern Virginia.

Shaunna Crossen, Ph.D., is an educational consultant with expertise in the areas of psychology, motivation and assessment. She received her B.S. from the University of Scranton and her M.A. and Ph.D. from the University of Delaware. Shaunna is an award-winning educator who has taught numerous undergraduate and graduate courses in education and psychology. She has consulted with corporations and served as the director of a statewide assessment program.

As an author, Shaunna has written several publications and research reports.
She resides in eastern Pennsylvania with her family.

You are about to begin an exciting journey into the world of cosmetology. The Certified Learning in Cosmetology® (CLiC) system will act as your road map, leading you to reap the rewards of becoming a successful professional cosmetologist.

The CLiC system is designed to enhance the fundamental cosmetology education by incorporating artistic inspiration and successful sales and retail skills. The learning modules cannot possibly cover all fashionable vogues, but will always encourage freedom of expression and innovation to adapt to current trends.

This revolutionary system focuses on meeting your educational needs with a solid, competency-based cosmetology curriculum. Each CLiC module is designed to develop manual dexterity, professional perception, tactile sensitivity and the artistic vision used in the field.

The CLiC educational system is presented in individual learning modules, each a complete program. The module system enables you to focus on individual disciplines within the field by offering courses for certified specialization in each field. This ensures the opportunity to learn and develop the skills needed for a rewarding and profitable career in the cosmetology field of your choice.

For additional information, contact:

CLiC INTERNATIONAL®
396 Pottsville/Saint Clair Highway
Pottsville, PA 17901 USA
1.800.207.5400 USA & Canada
001.570.429.4216 International
570.429.4252 Fax
info@clicusa.com
www.clicusa.com

CLiC INTERNATIONAL™

CERTIFIED LEARNING IN COSMETOLOGY®

CLiCer

Hello! My name is CLiCer (pronounced click-er), and I'm excited that you've joined me for this journey of learning in the field of cosmetology. I am joined by my partner Geno, to help show how people skills can directly and positively influence your success in the beauty business.

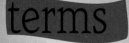

Terminology

To help reinforce your learning, terminology words appear highlighted throughout the book. This will help you recognize their importance at a glance. Definitions of these terms will be provided in Chapter One, the Visual Vocabulary. Chapter Seven will test you on these terms.

RA

Regulatory Alert

Whenever you see the **Regulatory Alert** icon, it will remind you and your instructor to check governmental regulations about the subject on the page. The rules and regulations for cosmetology vary according to geographic location. Your instructor will advise you of the regulations in your area.

CLiCer's Sales Pointers

Selling and financial skills will be just as important to your success in the salon as your actual technical knowledge and skills. Whenever you see this icon, pay special attention to the **sales pointers**. Combining sales skills with technical skills will create a dynamic force for your salon success.

Hello, I'm Geno! Since I can't be with you in the classroom, this image will take my place. My goal is to guide you through this book and add key ideas. When you see this image, pay close attention to what is said. "Geno-isms" will help you understand the importance of SUCCESS DYNAMICS and discover the art of people skills.

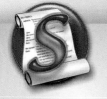

> READ THE WORD BALLOONS FOR DIALOGUE EXAMPLES.

Script

A script refers to rehearsed dialogue that is appropriate for specific situations. Throughout the book, you will find different types of scripts that should be memorized and practiced.
These scripts appear in purple. When you use scripts on a daily basis, they become a valuable communication tool.

Filmstrip Characters

Every day, you speak and interact with other people. But do you really think about what you are saying and how you are saying it? The importance of good dialogue skills in the beauty business cannot be emphasized enough. Pay close attention to the filmstrip dialogue to better understand the subject matter.

Awareness of your true potential in life is the greatest gift you can give yourself. Never underestimate the power of your brain and your ability to inspire creativity and facilitate the learning process.

The beauty business is one of the oldest professions known to the civilized world. During the days of the Pharaoh, pyramids were built with an area designed specifically for beauty artists. These beauty artists made sure that the Pharaoh and his family looked good when it was time to meet the gods.

Beauty professionals will always be in demand because people want to look their best, especially during important milestones in life. Before weddings, anniversaries, reunions, holidays, and other celebrations, clients flock to the salon to get polished, pampered and renewed.

There are so many career opportunities in the beauty industry for individuals who possess the necessary qualifications and the desire to provide excellent service. Take time to research the possibilities; seek information and ideas from respected professionals.

SUCCESS DYNAMICS is the foundation of your education and career in cosmetology. Success in the beauty industry depends on your ability to communicate effectively, promote positive relationships and market services and products.

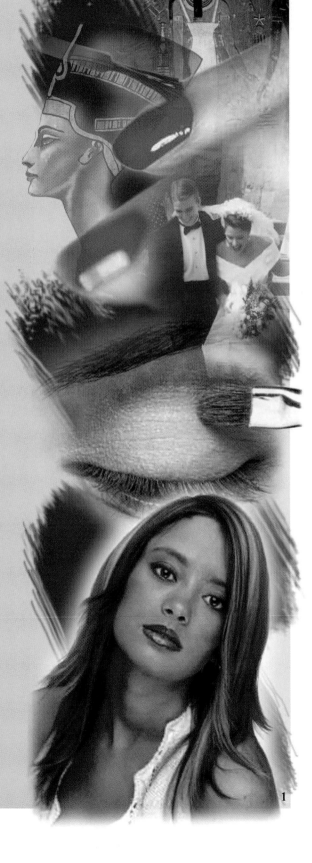

1

Table of Contents

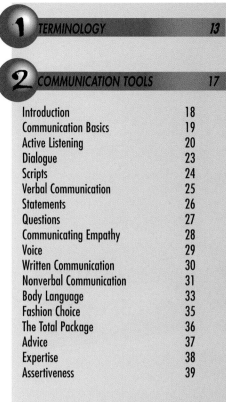

"For information about additional modules, check out the last page of this book."

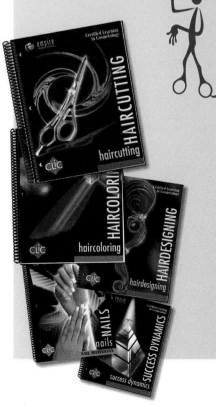

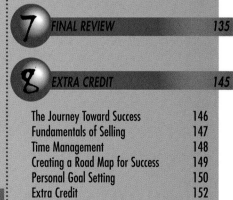

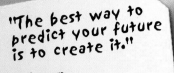

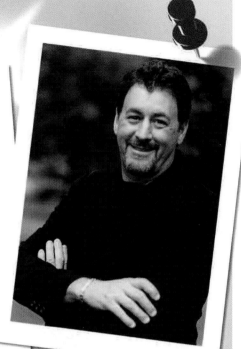

Dear Fellow Professional,

You may be wondering about the theme title of this book, On Stage. What does that mean? And more importantly, what's in this book for you? Let me share one of my guiding principles in life: "All the world is a stage." I believe that this quote by Shakespeare is absolutely true.

Each day, when you enter the salon or spa to work, you are stepping onto a stage. Whenever you conduct a consultation, perform a service, or even talk with others about what you do, you are on stage. It is your moment of truth, your opportunity to shine, to steal the show and create a memorable experience for every client that you serve.

Some clients are not familiar with the technical aspects of your job as a stylist; they judge your skills based on your ability to present yourself and provide excellent service. This book will guide you as you venture into the dynamic world of beauty.

The stage is set. The audience is eagerly awaiting your performance.

Be your best!
Geno Stampora

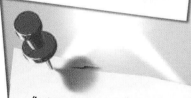

"Many of life's failures are people who did not realize how close they were to success when they gave up."

Thomas Edison
Inventor

"As professionals, we are always on stage, even when we're off stage."

Randy Rick
Creator of the CLiC Learning System

"Human beings, by changing inner attitudes of their minds, can change the outer aspects of their lives."

William James
Psychologist

"Man's mind, once stretched by a new idea, never regains its original dimensions."

Oliver Wendell Holmes, Jr.
US Supreme Court Justice

diversity
positioning
targeting
paraphrasing
revenue   stress
consultation

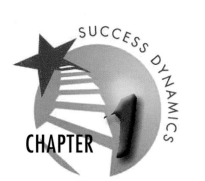

Terminology

TERMINOLOGY

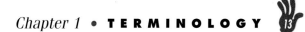

Terminology – A Visual Vocabulary

"Mastering the terminology of Success Dynamics is like learning a whole new language. It will give you the ability to communicate with future clients and fellow professionals. Your success starts here!"

Active Listening

Process by which the listener gives the speaker feedback about what was said.

Assertiveness

An honest, open expression of your thoughts and feelings.

Attitudes

Your own evaluation of the world around you.

Average Ticket Price (ATP)

A formula for determining how much the typical client pays for beauty services and products.

Body Language

Communication cues provided by the movement and position of your body.

Client Retention

Keeping existing clients.

Closed Question

Question that can be answered in a few words.

Consultation

The process of obtaining the information you need from the client in order to provide excellent service.

Discrimination

Unfair behavior directed toward members of another group.

Diversity

Distinct differences between people.

Emotional Intelligence

The ability to monitor your own and others' feelings and use this information to guide behavior.

Terminology ...

Finishing

Last phase of the service delivery model which begins with putting on the final touches and ends when the client leaves the salon.

Impression Management

Attempts to control how others perceive you.

Jargon

Words or phrases that only beauty industry professionals know.

Left-Brained

A term used to describe someone who performs well on verbal, analytical and logical tasks.

Marketing

The process of determining what customers need and then selling beauty services and products that satisfy those needs.

Networking

Utilizing social settings as an opportunity to meet new clients.

Nonverbal Communication

An unspoken language consisting of eye contact, facial expressions and body language.

Open Question

Question that invites the receiver to provide additional information.

Paraphrasing

Using your own words to summarize what you heard the speaker say.

Personality

An individual's unique combination of psychological characteristics and behavior patterns.

Personality Trait

Behavioral descriptor that explains the way people are in most situations.

Positioning

Process by which clients develop positive associations about their stylist and the salon.

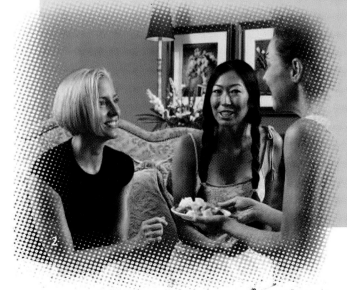

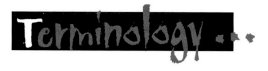
Prejudice

Unfair or negative attitude about another group.

Professionalism

Behaving in a manner appropriate for a business setting.

Rapport

Developing a close connection with someone you meet.

Revenue

Money earned from services provided.

Right-Brained

A term used to describe someone who performs well on visual, spatial and creative tasks.

Self-Actualization

The need to develop to your fullest potential.

Self-Esteem

An overall evaluation of your self-worth.

Slang

Informal words that are typically inappropriate for professionals to use.

Stereotype

Widely held belief about people who share a common trait or belong to particular group.

Stress

Physical and psychological responses to demanding situations.

Targeting

Directing marketing efforts toward those individuals who are most likely to purchase the service or product.

Up-Selling

Increasing the amount of money each customer spends on beauty services and products.

client retention
active listening
paraphrasing
jargon
open question
assertiveness
body language

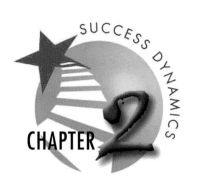

SUCCESS DYNAMICS
CHAPTER 2

Communication Tools

COMMUNICATION

GOALS

Keeping existing clients who come to you again and again is called client retention.

This chapter will help you communicate effectively. We begin with a discussion of communication goals and the three types of communication. Then we address specific situations where effective communication skills lead to more rewarding social interactions.

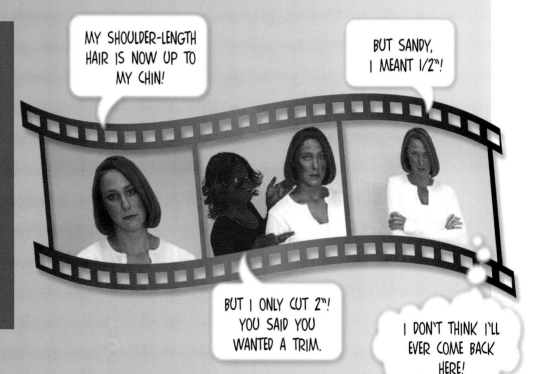

MY SHOULDER-LENGTH HAIR IS NOW UP TO MY CHIN!

BUT SANDY, I MEANT 1/2"!

BUT I ONLY CUT 2"! YOU SAID YOU WANTED A TRIM.

I DON'T THINK I'LL EVER COME BACK HERE!

"How well you communicate with clients will determine your success in the beauty industry."

By the time you complete this chapter, you should be able to:

- Use effective communication skills to improve your relationships.
- Follow the active listening model and increase your ability to understand others.
- Know how to ask questions to gain necessary information.
- Know how to read others by interpreting nonverbal cues.
- Understand conflict resolution strategies.

Communication Basics

With great communication tools, your career can skyrocket. Successful stylists listen to clients' concerns and solve their beauty problems.

Improve your ability to communicate by practicing the two fundamentals of great communication:

- **Listen to understand others.**
- **Speak using clear and specific words.**

GENO SAYS:
"Communication is an important tool beauty professionals use. It is just as important as your scissors, combs and brushes."

Communication is the process through which people exchange information. There are three goals of communication: to express, to understand, and to help others understand the information you give them.

Three Communication Goals (Long, 1996)

Goal	Sample Communication Exchange
To Express ○ Send messages that can be understood.	**Stylist:** *"To blow dry your hair with a round brush, you should…"*
To Understand ○ Accurately interpret others' messages.	**Client:** *"I don't want my fringes too short."* **Stylist:** *"I will cut your fringes while they are dry so I can make sure they fall slightly above your eyebrows."*
To Help Others Understand ○ Help others accurately interpret messages that you send.	**Stylist:** *"Adding highlights to your hair will add body and fullness. Highlights increase the thickness of the hair shaft, which creates volume."* **Client:** *"You think that highlights will give some life to my fine, limp hair? That sounds like a great idea!"*

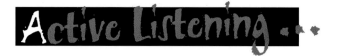

Active Listening ...

When communicating effectively, you will alternate between the role of sender and receiver. To do this, three types of communication are used: active listening, verbal communication, and nonverbal communication.

Active listening is the building block for all communication skills. During active listening, the listener gives the speaker feedback about what was said. This feedback takes the form of questions, interpretations, and clarifications *(Seta, 2000)*.

Four Steps to Active Listening:
(Fujishin, 2000)

1 FOCUS
Pay attention to and concentrate on the speaker.

2 SENSE
Use your eyes and ears to take in information.

3 UNDERSTAND
Comprehend what the speaker is saying and doing.

4 PARAPHRASE
Use your own words to summarize what you heard the speaker say.

FOCUS

SENSE

UNDERSTAND

PARAPHRASE

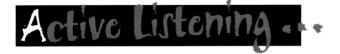

Active Listening ...

Active Listening requires the use of verbal and nonverbal (unspoken) signs that show the speaker you are interested in what he/she has to say *(Fujishin, 2000)*.

Verbal SIGNS of Active Listening

Nonverbal SIGNS of Active Listening

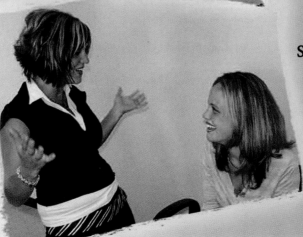

Avoid interrupting others.

Use direct eye contact, but don't stare for long periods of time.

Use encouragers:

"Oh."

"Mm-hmm."

"Okay."

"I see."

"Is that so?"

Occasionally nod your head.

Invite the speaker to share more information:

"Tell me more about it."

"I'm interested in your point of view."

Smile when appropriate.

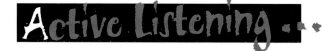

Active Listening...
PARAPHRASE

A critical component of active listening is paraphrasing because it shows the speaker that you understand the message. Paraphrasing is using your own words to summarize what you heard the speaker say.

Paraphrase by using the word "you" at the beginning of a statement.

Client: *"I really hate this drab color. Every strand of hair is the exact same shade of brown."*

Stylist: *"You probably feel that your hair is drab because there are no contrasting colors. Adding color would really add shine and texture to your hair. Let's discuss using a caramelizing effect on your hair."*

> I THINK I NEED A CHANGE. I'VE BEEN WEARING MY HAIR THE SAME WAY FOR TEN YEARS.

> YOU WOULD LIKE TO TRY A DIFFERENT LOOK.

> YES, I WOULD. WHAT DO YOU SUGGEST?

"Additional paraphrasing skills are discussed in Chapter Four."

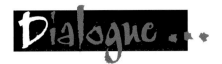

DIALOGUE

Dialogue refers to a communication exchange between two people.

In the beauty industry, the importance of effective dialogue cannot be underestimated.

Dialogue is used for all types of beauty services. Clients learn about your technical skills based on how well you explain each service.

Effective dialogue makes the difference between satisfactory service and excellent service.

If your car needed an oil change, which auto mechanic would you choose to service your car? At the first garage, the mechanic greets you by saying, *"What do you need?"* At the second garage, the mechanic offers the following greeting, *"Good morning. I'm looking forward to taking great care of your car today."*

2

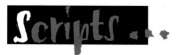

Scripts ...

Just as actors memorize lines before entering the stage, beauty professionals use scripts during every performance. A script refers to rehearsed dialogue that is appropriate for a specific situation.

Before conversing with clients, follow these recommendations to make scripts work for you.

RECOMMENDATIONS

- Set aside time to develop scripts.
- Practice scripts in front of the mirror and with others.
- Let the situation determine the script.

Throughout the book, you will find scripts that are appropriate for the various situations.

Types of Scripts

Networking

Greeting

Consultation

Finishing

Closing

Client complaints

Verbal Communication...

Verbal communication is sending a message using words. Have you ever had a misunderstanding because two people interpreted the same statement differently? Unfortunately, what the sender says is not always what the receiver hears. Therefore, use specific language when communicating.

In order to effectively communicate, avoid slang and jargon. Slang refers to informal words that are typically inappropriate for professionals to use. Jargon refers to words or phrases that only beauty industry professionals know.

SLANG

Incorrect: *"Ain't it great that you can use acrylic nails instead of waiting until your own nails grow?"*

Correct: *"Isn't it great..."*

Incorrect: *"Would you like to increase the level of your highlights?"*

Correct: *"Would you like to go a shade lighter with your highlights?"*

JARGON

Statements ...

Verbal communication consists of statements and questions. Statements are used to send messages.

When communicating, use three types of statements: expressive statements, summarizing statements, and empathetic responses *(Long, 1996)*.

Three Types of Statements

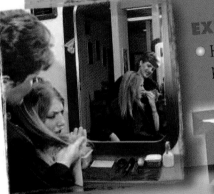

EXPRESSIVE STATEMENTS

- Help the client understand your point-of-view.

Dialogue Example:

"I recommend you use a conditioner once a week to replenish the moisture in your hair."

1

SUMMARIZING STATEMENTS

- Provide a summary of the main points to show the client that you accurately interpreted what she wants you to do.

Dialogue Example:

"What I heard you say is that you want a chin-length bob."

2

EMPATHETIC RESPONSES

- Show the client that you understand her thoughts or feelings by imagining yourself in her position.

Dialogue Example:

"It must have been very difficult to lose your hair during your illness."

3

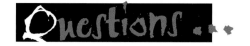
Questions are used to request information. "Closed" and "open" are the two main types of questions. Closed questions can be answered in a few words such as "yes" or "no." In comparison, open questions invite the receiver to provide additional information.

When communicating with shy or quiet clients, try using open questions to encourage them to talk. Instead of asking, *"Did you have a good day?"*, you will invite a more lengthy response by asking, *"What was your day like?"*

Two Types of Questions (Long, 1996)

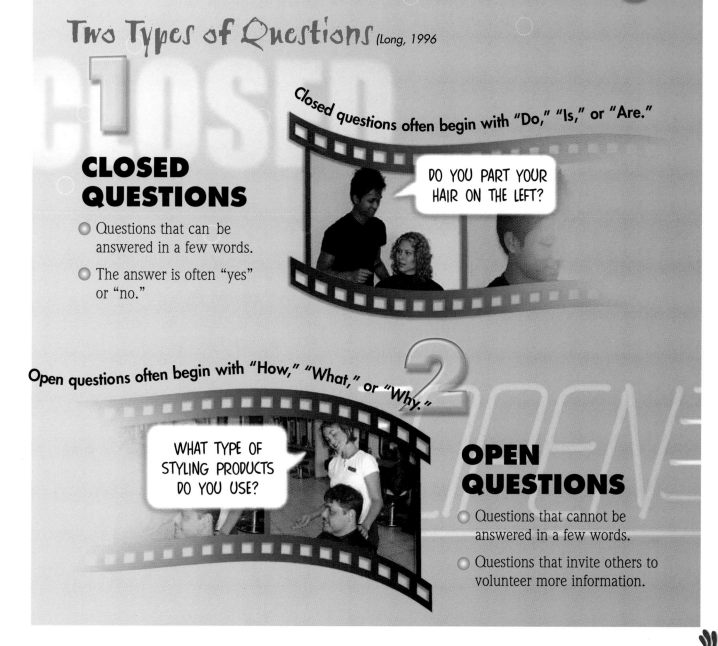

Closed questions often begin with "Do," "Is," or "Are."

CLOSED QUESTIONS

- Questions that can be answered in a few words.
- The answer is often "yes" or "no."

DO YOU PART YOUR HAIR ON THE LEFT?

Open questions often begin with "How," "What," or "Why."

WHAT TYPE OF STYLING PRODUCTS DO YOU USE?

OPEN QUESTIONS

- Questions that cannot be answered in a few words.
- Questions that invite others to volunteer more information.

Successful stylists connect with clients by using empathetic responses. When a client expresses a concern or complaint, you can convey empathy by using three critical words: feel, felt and found *(Katz, 1988)*.

Using "Feel," "Felt" and "Found"

Service Example

> I REALLY DON'T LIKE MY HAIR SHORT, BUT I THINK I SHOULD CUT IT. LONG HAIR DOESN'T SEEM TO LOOK RIGHT ON OLDER WOMEN.

> ASHLEY, I KNOW HOW YOU FEEL. THERE WERE TIMES I FELT LIKE THAT. I'VE FOUND THAT WITH THE PROPER CUT, MEDIUM-LENGTH HAIR LOOKS GREAT ON WOMEN OF ALL AGES.

Product Example

> I'D LIKE TO BUY THAT SHAMPOO, BUT IT SEEMS SO EXPENSIVE. THERE ARE SO MANY LESS EXPENSIVE PRODUCTS AVAILABLE IN THE GROCERY STORE.

> ERICA, I KNOW HOW YOU FEEL. I FELT LIKE THAT BEFORE I BECAME A STYLIST. I'VE FOUND THAT THE QUALITY OF PROFESSIONAL PRODUCTS MAKES THE RESULTS WORTH THE COST.

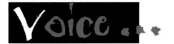
Voice ...

"Smiling before answering the phone helps to ensure a pleasant greeting."

When speaking with clients and coworkers, the way you sound is just as important as what you are saying. Use the characteristics of effective voice to enhance your communication skills.

Ineffective VOICE

- Jumbled sounds are difficult to understand.

- Talking too fast makes it difficult for the listener to follow the message.

  Talking too slowly causes others to feel impatient and frustrated.

- A high pitch can be annoying.

  A low pitch might be perceived as unapproachable.

- Monotone tends to be boring.

- We do not enjoy listening to people who speak too loudly or too softly.

Effective VOICE

Speak clearly.

Use an appropriate pace.

Use a pleasant pitch.

Use inflections in your voice.

Adjust your volume according to the environment.

Effective voice is particularly important when using the phone. Phone skills are needed to recruit clients, schedule appointments, and provide appointment reminders.

Written Communication...

Besides spoken communication, stylists also use written communication to send messages. Beauty professionals record information in appointment books, send thank you notes, and write home maintenance prescriptions.

Home Maintenance Personal Prescription

FOR _____

STYLIST _____

SHAMPOO _____

CONDITIONER _____

STYLING AIDS _____

FINISHING PRODUCT _____

Thank You!

WRITING STRATEGIES

- Visualize others reading what you are writing.
- Take the time to write neatly. Make sure that others can read your handwriting.
- Keep notes and messages short and to the point.
- Be polite. Remember to thank clients and sign your name to notes and prescriptions.

Nonverbal Communication...

Nonverbal communication is an unspoken language consisting of eye contact, facial expressions and body language. Compared to verbal communication, nonverbal communication is more difficult to control.

Even when people try to hide their feelings, emotions are often expressed through nonverbal cues *(DePaulo, 1992)*. For instance, parents often detect when their young children are lying because most adults know that it is difficult to lie when looking directly into someone's eyes.

1

2

Eye Contact

Beliefs about appropriate eye contact vary across cultures. For most people who identify with Western cultures, eye contact is a sign of respect. We show that we care about what is being said by looking directly into the speaker's eyes. When people avoid eye contact, they are often viewed as unfriendly or shy *(Zimbardo, 1977)*.

Facial Expressions

In addition to observing people's eyes, we also gather important information by interpreting facial expressions. Smiling, frowning, and eyebrow raising are types of facial expressions. These expressions are combined to communicate different thoughts or emotions. Researchers have estimated that there are at least 640 different facial expressions *(Fujishin, 2000).*

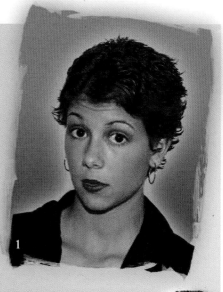

Smiling is a universally recognized expression. People who smile are viewed as happy, attractive, sociable, sincere and competent *(Reis et al., 1990).*

GENO SAYS:

"Many times people tell you more with actions than words. Learn to read nonverbal signs."

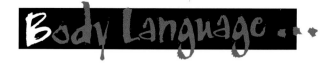 Body Language ...

Body language refers to communication cues that are provided by the movement and position of your body. These signals provide information about your emotional state.

When observing people's body movements, ask yourself:

○ How much is their body moving?

○ Which body parts are moving?

Posture

Did you ever hear an adult tell a child to stand up straight? Besides helping to ensure good body alignment, an erect posture communicates that you are a confident person.

Movement

A still body suggests that the individual is in a relaxed state. In comparison, considerable body movements, such as rubbing or scratching, suggest impatience or nervousness.

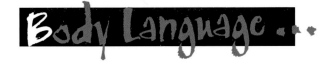
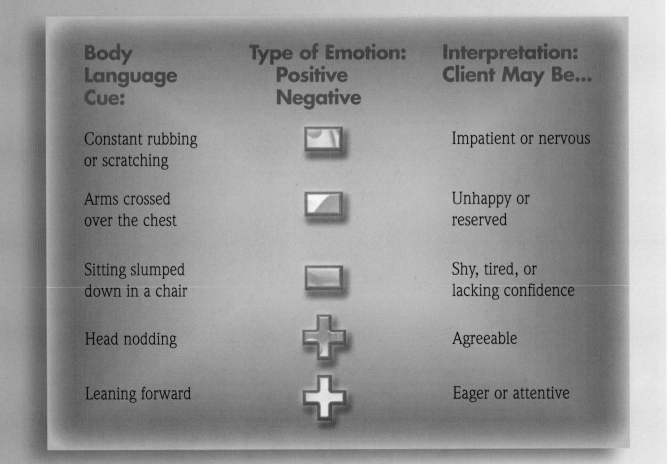

"Watch that bubble!"

intimate space - 0" to 18"

Proximity refers to the degree of physical space between individuals. *Hall (1990)* defined the boundary of intimate space as 0 to 18 inches (0 cm to 46 cm). This is often referred to as your "personal bubble," which is reserved for activities such as hugging or holding intimate conversations.

Working as a stylist requires you to be within your client's personal bubble. Some clients might feel a bit uncomfortable experiencing such physical closeness. Be mindful of nonverbal cues that might signal discomfort, such as a client who pulls her body away from you.

Body Language Cue:	Type of Emotion: Positive Negative	Interpretation: Client May Be...
Constant rubbing or scratching		Impatient or nervous
Arms crossed over the chest		Unhappy or reserved
Sitting slumped down in a chair		Shy, tired, or lacking confidence
Head nodding		Agreeable
Leaning forward		Eager or attentive

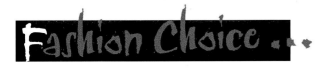

Fashion Choice...

While working in a salon, it is important to make the distinction between personal fashion statement and fashion choice.

Your personal fashion statement may be jeans and a t-shirt, but this might not be acceptable in a successful salon environment. Likewise, piercings and tattoos may be offensive to some clients.

Successful stylists pay close attention to their fashion choices, especially while at work. Why take a fashion risk that could cost you clients?

"Use good judgment in selecting professional attire that is comfortable and flexible."

Personal Fashion Statement at Home

Jeans, t-shirt
Old, dirty sneakers
Nose and belly button rings
Tattoos

Fashion Choice at Work

Dress pants, blouse
Clean, shiny shoes
No piercings
No visible tattoos

RA

Check with your regulatory authority for approved professional attire.

The Total Package ...

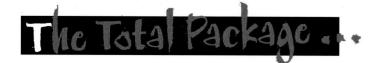

Image

Even while silent, you communicate through your actions and appearance. The way you dress tells others a great deal of information about you. Based on style of dress, people make judgments about your personality, technical skills and level of success.

Geno Says:
"Always imagine yourself on stage whenever you are in public. Present a professional image that communicates confidence in yourself and your abilities."

You are a walking advertisement for your services. Therefore, it is critical to always look your best. If you dress like a professional and your hairstyle is trendy, clients will be more likely to seek your services to achieve an updated look for themselves.

"Additional recommendations about dressing for success are presented in Chapter Six."

Appearance — **Negative Impression**

Wrinkled or faded clothes

Messy hair

Too much makeup

"My stylist . . .
. . . is sloppy and careless."
. . . pays little attention to detail."
. . . lacks beauty sense."

Appearance — **Positive Impression**

Fashionable clothes

Trendy hairstyle

Flawless makeup and nails

"My stylist . . .
. . . has an updated fashion sense."
. . . knows current beauty trends."
. . . is an all-around beauty expert."

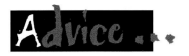

Rules for Giving Advice

Stylists are paid to offer advice. Follow these rules to maximize the benefits of giving advice.

3 "BE"

RA

Remember, limit your advice to products and services! Depending on your location, any other advice may be against the law.

BE Knowledgeable

People are more likely to follow the advice of an expert than a non-expert *(Baron & Byrne, 2002)*. For this reason, many commercials show experts selling products. Knowledge of services and products helps you maintain expert status.

BE Sincere

Many clients are aware that stylists receive a commission for selling beauty products. Recommend services and products that you believe will result in personal improvements for clients. Suggestions that are perceived to be based on selfish motives will decrease client retention.

BE Proactive

Record your recommendations and list the purchased services and products on each client's record card. During the next consultation, ask follow-up questions to determine whether the client was satisfied.

When suggesting a service or product, focus on specific benefits for the client.

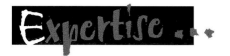

Your success in the beauty industry depends on achieving expert status.

Importance of Being Perceived as a Beauty Expert

1 If clients view you as an expert, they will be less likely to look for another stylist.

2 Experts are more persuasive than non-experts when selling services and products.

3 Coworkers will respect and value your opinion if they view you as an expert.

Service professionals are people who are in the business of helping others. Think of a service professional who you consider an expert. Are you thinking of a doctor, teacher, stylist, or some other professional? How would you describe this person to a stranger?

It is unlikely that your description would include shy, quiet, or hesitant to state his or her opinion. Rather, you would describe an expert as honest, outgoing and confident about his or her ability to help others.

> I HAVE TO DISAGREE WITH YOU. I REALLY BELIEVE THAT STAYING OPEN UNTIL 9:30 AT NIGHT WILL BRING MORE CLIENTS TO THE SALON.

Assertiveness is an honest, open expression of your thoughts and feelings. Assertive people respectfully express their opinions, even if they disagree with what others are thinking or saying *(Dickson, Hargie, & Morrow, 1989)*.

People who lack assertiveness often fail to speak up because they are concerned about what others will think. On the other hand, some people take assertiveness too far and are perceived as aggressive or disrespectful. There are key components of assertiveness that will help you maintain professional status.

Components of Assertiveness

- ◎ Respect others' thoughts and feelings.
- ◎ Communicate your views in an honest, open manner.
- ◎ Speak with confidence.
- ◎ Believe that what you have to say is important.

> ADDING SOME HIGHLIGHTS AROUND YOUR FACE WILL REALLY BRING OUT YOUR EYE COLOR.

Assertiveness

In addition to promoting positive relationships, assertiveness can also be used to address conflicts when they arise.

"Carefully choose the time and place to speak your mind."

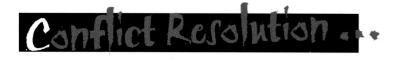

Conflict Resolution ...

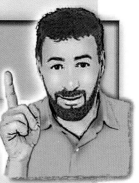

Geno Says:
"Never talk down to clients or coworkers."

Conflicts, also known as disagreements, are an inevitable part of life. It is unrealistic to believe that you will never have conflicts with clients or coworkers. Unfortunately, when you do not appropriately resolve conflicts, there can be negative consequences. You risk losing clients, support from coworkers and possibly even your job.

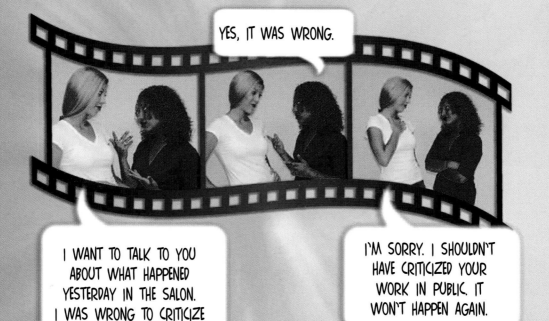

YES, IT WAS WRONG.

I WANT TO TALK TO YOU ABOUT WHAT HAPPENED YESTERDAY IN THE SALON. I WAS WRONG TO CRITICIZE YOUR CLIENT'S HAIRCUT.

I'M SORRY. I SHOULDN'T HAVE CRITICIZED YOUR WORK IN PUBLIC. IT WON'T HAPPEN AGAIN.

Follow a simple childhood rule:

I'm Sorry

Say *"I'm sorry,"* when you do something that hurts someone else's feelings.

Focus on your own feelings. Don't blame others.

The most important rule of conflict resolution is to own your feelings. Avoid blaming someone else for making you feel a certain way. Placing blame causes others to be defensive and put up additional barriers.

Learning how to communicate effectively includes controlling your emotions. People who speak with their emotions when they are angry, hurt, or upset usually end up offending others.

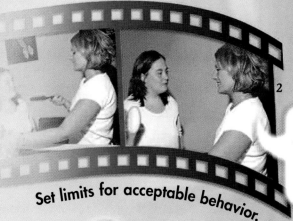

> YESTERDAY, I WAS REALLY UPSET BECAUSE I FELT EMBARRASSED IN FRONT OF MY COWORKERS.

> I WOULD LIKE TO DISCUSS WHAT MADE YOU SO ANGRY, BUT I WILL NOT ALLOW YOU TO YELL AT ME.

Set limits for acceptable behavior.

Strategies

Conflict Resolution Strategies
(Weiten, 2002)

- Address the conflict directly. Do not avoid the person or refuse to speak to him/her.
- Remain calm. Speak using a normal tone of voice.
- Focus on your own feelings. Avoid blaming others.
- Set limits for acceptable behavior.
- Express your willingness to compromise.

> I'D LIKE TO COME UP WITH A SOLUTION THAT WORKS FOR BOTH OF US.

Express your willingness to compromise.

To communicate more clearly, consider practicing every day. Successful beauty professionals continually work on their dialogue and communication skills. Ask yourself the following reflection questions and use your responses to develop an Action Plan.

Set aside time each day to reflect on your experiences by focusing on:

- what worked well,
- what did not work, and
- how to improve your business.

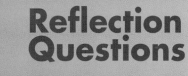

Reflection Questions	Communication Action Plan
	I will...
How can I communicate my message to others?	use specific words, avoid slang and jargon.
	use body language cues that communicate positive emotions.
Am I asking appropriate questions?	use open questions when I want the client to share a lot of information.
	use closed questions when I want the client to give a brief response.

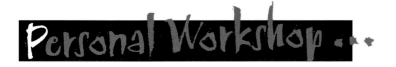

Ask yourself the following reflection questions and use your responses to develop an Action Plan.

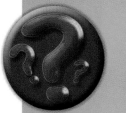

Reflection Questions

Communication Action Plan

I will...

How can I encourage clients to express themselves?

follow the active listening model: focus, sense, understand, and paraphrase.

connect with clients by using empathetic responses.

What must I do to appear more confident as a communicator?

dress professionally while at work.

be assertive by expressing my views in an honest, open manner.

choose an appropriate time to express myself.

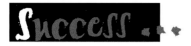

The elements of successful communication and professional relationships can be remembered as follows:

Self-Awareness

is learning about who you are and what stresses you, how you feel about yourself and how you come across to others.

Understanding

is the ability to use listening and communication skills to see another person's situation from that person's point of view.

Competence

is achieved when the skills and techniques in this book are mastered and have become a part of how you interact with others.

Compassion

is understanding the needs of others.

Emotional Health

is making sure that stress reduction and coping skills are part of your daily life.

Style

is your talents and personality combined with what you learn from your teachers and mentors.

Self-Confidence

is a result of the ongoing experience of putting all these skills into practice and knowing that YOU CAN DO IT.

Printed with permission from Mildred Gordon, Ph.D.

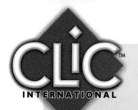

Communication Tools REVIEW QUESTIONS

MATCHING

F **1.** Words or phrases that only beauty professionals know.

B **2.** An honest, open expression of your thoughts and feelings.

A **3.** Process by which the listener gives the speaker feedback about what was said.

GA **4.** Communication cues provided by the movement and position of your body.

C **5.** An unspoken language consisting of eye contact, facial expressions, and body language.

H **6.** Question that invites the receiver to provide additional information.

J **7.** Informal words that are typically inappropriate for professionals to use.

I **8.** Using your own words to summarize what you heard the speaker say.

E **9.** Question that can be answered in a few words.

D **10.** Keeping existing clients.

A. Active Listening
B. Assertiveness
C. Body Language
D. Client Retention
E. Closed Question
F. Jargon
G. Nonverbal Communication
H. Open Question
I. Paraphrasing
J. Slang

TYPES OF STATEMENTS

Use the following key to identify each statement:
P = Paraphrase
E = Empathetic Response

11. P *"It sounds like you are very unhappy with your current hairstyle."*

12. P *"You think that shorter hair would make your face look slimmer."*

13. E *"I can only imagine how difficult it must be to care for someone with a terminal illness."*

14. P *"I hear you saying that you want your highlights to be a shade lighter than your natural color."*

15. E *"It must seem like time passes so slowly when you're waiting for bangs to grow out."*

OPEN & CLOSED QUESTIONS

Use the following key to identify each question:
O = Open
C = Closed

16. O *"How do you like living on the East Coast?"*

17. C *"Do you use conditioner every day?"*

18. O *"What do you like to do during your free time?"*

19. C *"Is your hair naturally wavy?"*

20. C *"Would you like something to drink?"*

STUDENT'S NAME   DATE   GRADE

GET TO THE POINT
By K. Berg and A. Gilman
Bantam; New York, 1989

THE FIRST FIVE MINUTES
By N. King
Prentice Hall; New York, 1987

SMART QUESTIONS
By D. Leeds
Berkley Books; New York, 1987

HOW TO COMMUNICATE
By J. McKay, M. Davis and P. Fanning
MJF Books; New York, 1983

POWER SPEAKING
By M. Yarnell and K.B. McCommon
VCA Books; Evanston, IL, 1987

prejudice
attitudes
personality
discrimination
self-esteem
diversity
stereotype

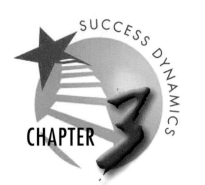

Science of Understanding People

UNDERSTANDING PEOPLE

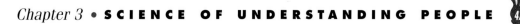

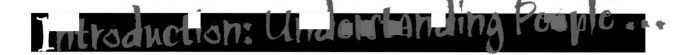

Understanding people is critical for success in the beauty industry. Most industry experts believe in the "80-20" formula for success. That is, 80% of salon success results from excellent people skills, whereas 20% stems from superb technical skills.

This chapter will help you interact more effectively with clients and coworkers.

This chapter begins with a focus on understanding yourself. Then, we examine approaches to interacting with different personalities and working as a team. Finally, we address the importance of respecting differences.

By the time you complete this chapter, you should be able to:

- Describe behaviors that convey positive and negative attitudes.
- Understand the relationship between goal setting and high self-esteem.
- Use Maslow's Hierarchy of Needs to understand client cancellations and "no-shows."
- Describe strategies for working with difficult personalities.
- Understand how to eliminate prejudice and discrimination when interacting with people.

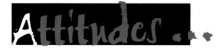

Attitudes ...

Attitude Component	EXAMPLE: Women Who Wear Makeup

Success in the beauty industry depends on conveying a positive attitude that attracts others to you. Attitudes represent your evaluations of the world. These evaluations may be positive, negative or neutral (neutral is neither positive nor negative).

Many stylists believe that women are more attractive when they wear makeup. Using this example, we will explain the three components of an attitude: belief, emotion and action *(Coon, 2003)*.

Successful stylists rely on these three attitude components to appear positive and upbeat even when feeling angry, sick or upset.

BELIEF — Wearing makeup improves a woman's appearance.

EMOTION — I feel more attractive when wearing makeup.

ACTION — I take time to buy cosmetics so that I can apply makeup every day.

Clients are more likely to seek beauty services from a stylist who displays a positive attitude.

Behaviors That Convey A Positive Attitude	Behaviors That Convey A Negative Attitude
✚ Smiling	▬ Frowning
✚ Offering praise for genuine accomplishments	▬ Criticizing
✚ Using sincere compliments	▬ Providing negative evaluations or insults
✚ Respecting others	▬ Gossiping or lying
✚ Offering congratulations	▬ Belittling someone's accomplishments
✚ Displaying a positive outlook on life	▬ Displaying a negative outlook on life

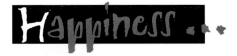

Happiness is a choice. Unfortunately, some people believe they do not have control of their own attitude. As a result, they allow events in their lives and people around them to affect their attitude.

One technique for sustaining happiness is to visualize a horizontal line that separates positive and negative attitudes. Maintain a positive attitude by bringing negative events and negative people up to the positive side of the line. This approach will help prevent others from controlling your mood.

When a client conveys a negative attitude you can express disagreement without being argumentative, as shown in the following examples:

POSITIVE ATTITUDE

NEGATIVE ATTITUDE

I GUESS EVERYONE IS ENTITLED TO THEIR OWN OPINION ABOUT WHAT LOOKS GOOD.

ONE THING I'VE LEARNED FROM WORKING IN A SALON IS THAT EVERYONE HAS THEIR OWN IDEAS ABOUT WHAT IS BEAUTIFUL.

WHY WOULD ANYONE WANT PAINTED PICTURES ON THEIR BODY? TATTOOS ARE GROSS.

BODY PIERCING IS UGLY. I DON'T UNDERSTAND WHY PEOPLE PUT HOLES IN THEIR BODY.

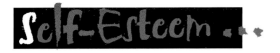

Self-Esteem ...

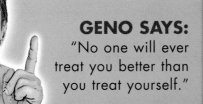

GENO SAYS:
"No one will ever treat you better than you treat yourself."

HIGH SELF-ESTEEM

Besides attitudes, people also possess an overall evaluation of their self-worth as either high or low. This is called self-esteem.

Self-esteem is based on how you see yourself in specific areas, such as: physical appearance, relationships, academics and job performance *(Harter, 1999)*.

Studies have shown that compared to people with low self-esteem, individuals with high self-esteem are more motivated and productive at work *(e.g., Mossholder, Bedeian & Armenakis, 1982)*.

Fortunately, a person's self-esteem is subject to change based on new experiences and information *(Markus & Nurius, 1986)*. One way to increase self-esteem is to read books about others who have overcome life's challenges in order to succeed. For example, consider reading about Abraham Lincoln and everything he did to achieve his goal of becoming President of the United States.

Another way to increase self-esteem is through goal setting. Self-esteem grows when you set realistic, but challenging goals and work hard to meet those goals.

Goal Setting: Key to High Self-Esteem *(Brophy, 1988)*

STRATEGY	EXAMPLE
Set reasonable but challenging goals for yourself.	*"I'm going to bring in five new clients next week."*
Realistically take credit for your successes.	*"By using my contacts and good social skills, I was able to meet my goal."*
View failure as providing important feedback about how to improve.	*"I wasn't able to reach my goal because I didn't…"*
Recognize when failure occurs due to factors outside of your control.	*"Unfortunately, I wasn't able to meet my goal because three of the five new clients were 'no-shows.'"*

For some people, low self-esteem stems from the belief that they are not smart. In this case, the path to improved self-esteem can be found by recognizing that intelligence is more than just "book smarts."

"Additional information about goal setting is presented in Chapter Eight."

Emotional Intelligence...

People who are in the business of helping others must rely on Emotional Intelligence (EI) to best serve their clients. EI consists of the ability to monitor your own and others' feelings and use that information to guide behavior *(Salovey & Mayer, 1990)*. According to *Goleman (2001)*, EI incorporates a variety of people skills including:

EMPATHY

CONFIDENCE

COMMUNICATION

EMOTIONAL SELF-CONTROL

CONFLICT MANAGEMENT

TEAMWORK

"All of these skills are addressed in this book because effective people skills are critical for success in the beauty industry."

Successful stylists use EI to show clients that they are sensitive and caring. One way to do this is by maintaining emotional self-control at all times.

Example:
While shampooing your client's hair, she described her neighbor in prejudicial terms. You were offended by her choice of words, but wanted to show professionalism.

Stylist:
"I'm really not comfortable using that term. I prefer to use..."

GENO SAYS:
"Pamper and respect every client."

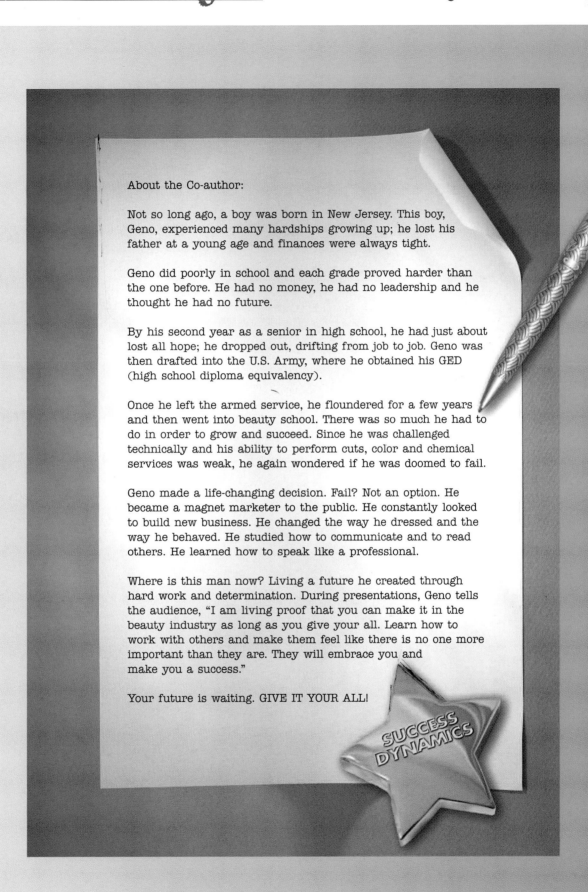

About the Co-author:

Not so long ago, a boy was born in New Jersey. This boy, Geno, experienced many hardships growing up; he lost his father at a young age and finances were always tight.

Geno did poorly in school and each grade proved harder than the one before. He had no money, he had no leadership and he thought he had no future.

By his second year as a senior in high school, he had just about lost all hope; he dropped out, drifting from job to job. Geno was then drafted into the U.S. Army, where he obtained his GED (high school diploma equivalency).

Once he left the armed service, he floundered for a few years and then went into beauty school. There was so much he had to do in order to grow and succeed. Since he was challenged technically and his ability to perform cuts, color and chemical services was weak, he again wondered if he was doomed to fail.

Geno made a life-changing decision. Fail? Not an option. He became a magnet marketer to the public. He constantly looked to build new business. He changed the way he dressed and the way he behaved. He studied how to communicate and to read others. He learned how to speak like a professional.

Where is this man now? Living a future he created through hard work and determination. During presentations, Geno tells the audience, "I am living proof that you can make it in the beauty industry as long as you give your all. Learn how to work with others and make them feel like there is no one more important than they are. They will embrace you and make you a success."

Your future is waiting. GIVE IT YOUR ALL!

SUCCESS DYNAMICS

Maslow's (1970) Hierarchy of Needs provides a framework to understand human behavior. According to Maslow, life is a journey to satisfy five types of needs. The ultimate need is self-actualization, which is the need to develop to your full potential. In other words, self-actualization is the desire to be all that you can be.

Maslow used a hierarchy, a model shaped like a pyramid, to show the relationship between basic survival needs and other higher level needs. He argued that you are first motivated to satisfy basic survival and safety needs. Once these needs are met, you can work your way toward self-actualization.

1 Individuals must first satisfy basic *biological needs* for food, water and sleep.

2 We are then motivated to satisfy *safety needs* including protection from harm.

3 Next we are driven to satisfy the *need to love and feel a sense of belonging*.

4 This is followed by *esteem needs* which include achieving goals, gaining approval and obtaining recognition.

5 After all of these needs are met, the *need for self-actualization* takes over, which is striving to achieve your unique potential.

Self-Actualization

The need to find out who you are and develop to your fullest potential

Esteem Needs — Need for self-respect & the respect of others

Love & Belonging Needs — Need for love, affection, & a sense of belonging

Safety Needs — Need for security, & freedom from fear

Biological Needs — Need for water, food & sleep

The Hierarchy of Needs is particularly helpful when trying to understand client cancellations. Sometimes, there are legitimate client needs and priorities that interfere with appointments. In these situations, empathetic responses work well because they help you connect with clients and show them that you care.

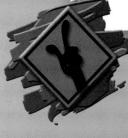

Call clients to remind them of upcoming appointments.

Application of Maslow's Hierarchy of Needs
Problem: Client Cancellations

Example

Jonathan, a successful businessman, worked fifteen hours. He was so wrapped up in his work that he forgot about his appointment.

Kathy missed her perm appointment because she was pleading with her boyfriend not to call off their engagement.

Since taking her new medication, Mrs. Francis has been experiencing fainting spells and is afraid to drive.

Empathetic Response

"Jonathan, I understand that your job is very demanding. Would you like our receptionist to e-mail you a reminder?"

"Kathy, please don't feel badly . There were so many walk-ins, I did three haircuts during your appointment time."

"Mrs. Francis, I would never expect you to risk your life to come for a hair appointment!"

Esteem Needs

Love and Belonging Needs

Safety Needs

Biological Needs

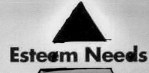

EMPATHY

Competence
Competence
Competence
Competence

Flexibility

Warmth

Personality is what makes each of us different. Personality consists of a person's unique combination of psychological characteristics and behavior patterns.

Successful beauty professionals learn how to work with a chameleon personality. This gives them the ability to converse with clients from all walks of life and make clients feel good about themselves.

If asked to describe your favorite stylist, you might respond by using adjectives, such as friendly, honest, funny and energetic. These personality traits are behavioral descriptors that explain the way people are in most situations. In general, successful stylists share three personality traits: flexibility, warmth and competence.

Personality Traits of Successful Stylists

TRAIT BEHAVIORS

Flexibility
- Adapt easily to new situations and different types of people.

Warmth
- Display a genuine, positive attitude.
- Speak kindly of others. "She's a lovely person."
- Demonstrate great conversation skills.

Competence
- Listen actively.
- Speak with confidence.
- Provide clear explanations.

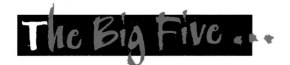

The Big Five ...

When trying to understand others, it is helpful to apply the Big Five personality model from the field of psychology.

The Big Five refers to five traits that usually remain constant during a person's adulthood *(Costa & McCrae, 1987).*

People's intensity level on each trait ranges from high to low.

Knowing your intensity level will improve your interactions with others. In general, it is easier to relate to clients who are similar to yourself.

THE BIG FIVE PERSONALITY TRAITS

DIMENSION	INTENSITY	BEHAVIORS
Openness to Experience	**HIGH** Adventurous, curious, imaginative	**Willing to try different styles or services**
	LOW Conservative	Prefer same hair styles or conventional styles
Conscientiousness	**HIGH** Dependable, determined, organized	**On time, hard working, concerned about appearance**
	LOW Unreliable, late	Forget appointments, late for appointments
Extroversion	**HIGH** Outgoing, assertive, energetic	**Great conversationalist, good listener**
	LOW Introverted, reserved, passive	Quiet, difficult to get to know
Agreeableness	**HIGH** Easy-going, cooperative, helpful, trusting	**Understanding if you're running behind schedule**
	LOW Critical, irritable	Unhappy with delays, difficult to please
Neuroticism	**HIGH** Insecure, depressed, anxious	**Emotional, moody**
	LOW Calm, even-tempered	Comfortable, unemotional

Adapted from Costa & McCrae (1987)

Researchers have found that most individuals can be categorized as displaying either the Type A or Type B personality. Compared to the Type A personality, the Type B personality is calm, unhurried and non-competitive *(Friedman & Rosenman, 1974).*

Type A Personality		Strategies for Working with Type A Clients
Characteristic	**Behaviors**	
Impatient with delay	Fidgeting in seat Looking at watch	○ Be mindful of the time. ○ Work quickly and efficiently. ○ Spend less time on finishing touches.
Explosive or accelerated speech	Speaking quickly and loudly Displaying anger	○ Speak slowly in a soft voice.
Competitive	Striving for success Challenging others	○ Offer praise for the individual's accomplishments.

Type B Personality		Strategies for Working with Type B Clients
Characteristic	**Behaviors**	
Calm and unhurried	Sitting still in a relaxed state	○ If you have time before the next appointment, show the client several styling options.
Non-competitive	Working cooperatively	○ Praise the individual for his/her ability to work well with others.

Adapted from Friedman & Rosenman (1974)

GENO SAYS: "Give consistent value to every client."

Undoubtedly, you will encounter both Type A and B personalities. Research has indicated that approximately 40% of the population display the Type A personality and 60% show the Type B personality *(Seta, Paulus & Baron, 2000).*

Difficult Personalities ...

Stylists work with a range of client personalities. Most clients are extroverted and agreeable. However, you will work with some clients who are difficult. The following table presents strategies for working with five types of difficult clients.

TYPE OF CLIENT	CHARACTERISTIC	STRATEGIES
Hostile-aggressive	Difficult to please Argumentative	Speak in a calm voice.
Complainers/ Negativists	Constant unhappiness Always upset about a problem	Acknowledge gripes. Listen to problems.
Silent and unresponsive	Introverted personality	Use open-ended questions to encourage dialogue.
Know-it-all Experts	Think they know more than everyone else	Praise them for their accomplishments. Ask for their opinion/advice.
Indecisives	Cannot make a decision	Present several options and give recommendations.

Adapted from Bramson (1987)

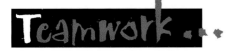

Your coworkers are a team of professionals who work together to provide the best beauty services. A great team leaves a positive, lasting impression on clients.

The essence of teamwork is learning how to bring out the best in one other. Look for these key qualities in yourself and others: care, cooperation and respect.

Fundamentals of a Great Team Player

1 Always support your fellow teammates.

2 Make your salon a happy place to work.

3 Work with and grow from your mentors.

4 Focus on work while at work and school while at school.

5 Give others room to be themselves.

Essential Components of Teamwork

COMPONENT	DESCRIPTION
CARE	Help coworkers do their jobs better. Offer constructive criticism. Provide emotional support.
COOPERATION	Put customers first. Work together to achieve common goals. Share credit and knowledge.
RESPECT	Accept and celebrate differences. Be open to other points of view. Develop an atmosphere of mutual respect.

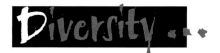

An important part of working with people

is understanding diversity. Diversity refers to distinct differences between people. There are many ways in which people differ including age, race, sexual preference, income and appearance.

Three important terms related to diversity are stereotype, prejudice and discrimination.

TERM	DEFINITION	EXAMPLES
STEREOTYPE	Widely held **belief** about people who share a common trait or belong to a particular group.	*"People with blonde hair are stupid."*
PREJUDICE	**Unfair or negative attitude** about another group.	*"I do not like to work with blondes because they are stupid."*
DISCRIMINATION	**Unfair behavior** directed toward members of another group.	*"I refuse to accept blondes as clients because they are stupid."*

Adapted from Plotnik (2002)

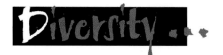

Some people are unaware that they communicate prejudicial attitudes when using specific words and phrases. The table below describes ways to eliminate prejudice and discrimination when communicating.

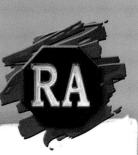

Signed in 1990, the Americans with Disabilities Act (ADA) guarantees that people with disabilities have access to all public services. It is against the law to deny beauty services to them.

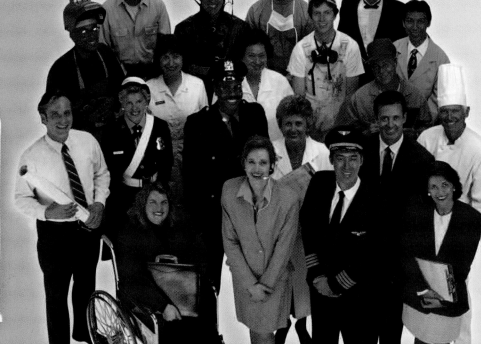

Eliminating Prejudice and Discrimination When Communicating

TOPIC	STRATEGY	SOCIALLY ACCEPTABLE TERM
Occupations	Use gender-neutral language.	Flight attendant Mail carrier Police officer Server
People with Disabilities	Replace the word "handicap."	Disability
Ethnic and Racial Differences	Avoid ethnic or racial slurs.	Latino African-American Caucasian
Differences in Sexual Orientation	Avoid derogatory terms.	Gay Lesbian

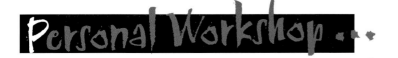

The key to self-enhancement is to create time everyday to fine tune your attitude. Ask yourself the following reflection questions and use your responses to develop an Action Plan.

Reflection Questions	Positive Attitide Action Plan
	I will ...
What can I incorporate into my personality to become more attractive to others?	display a positive attitude. maintain emotional self-control.
How can I become aware of my true and complete potential?	set realistic, but challenging goals. view failure as providing important feedback.
How can I earn the trust of others?	avoid gossiping. speak kindly of others.
What can I do to become a more valued team player?	support my coworkers. offer praise for accomplishments.

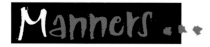

Having good manners is an essential component of salon etiquette. Clients may choose not to work with professionals who appear rude or ignorant. Be mindful of "salon manners."

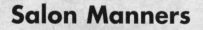

Salon Manners

- Be polite.
- Thank clients for their business.
- Wash hands after eating, smoking or using the lavatory.
- Avoid chewing gum.
- Make sure clients are comfortable. Treat clients as you would treat guests in your home.
- Say "excuse me" if you interrupt others.
- Say "pardon me" when asking someone to repeat statements that you did not hear.

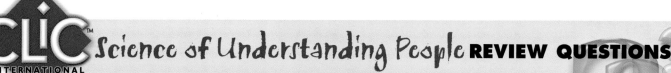

MATCHING

J **1.** Widely held belief about people who share a common trait or belong to a particular group.

G **2.** Unfair behavior directed toward members of another group.

A **3.** Your evaluation of the world around you.

X **4.** An individual's unique and relatively unchanging psychological characteristics and behavior patterns.

D **5.** The ability to monitor your own and others' feelings and use this information to guide behavior.

IX **6.** An overall evaluation of your self-worth.

B **7.** Unfair or negative attitude about another group.

E **8.** Behavioral descriptors that explain the way you are in most situations.

H **9.** The need to develop to your fullest potential.

C **10.** The distinct differences between people.

A. Attitudes
B. Discrimination
C. Diversity
D. Emotional Intelligence
E. Personality
F. Personality Traits
G. Prejudice
H. Self-Actualization
I. Self-Esteem
J. Stereotype

TRUE OR FALSE

T **1.** Three components of an attitude are: belief, emotion and action.

F **2.** A person's self-esteem never changes.

F **3.** All people who have "book smarts" are also emotionally intelligent.

T **4.** According to Maslow's Hierarchy of Needs, the ultimate need is to feel a sense of belonging.

T **5.** It is against the law to deny beauty services to individuals because they have a disability.

T **6.** Safety needs include the need for self-respect.

F **7.** The best way to handle a hostile client is to raise your voice.

T **8.** If a client is Type A personality, you should take extra time to chat while performing salon services.

T **9.** The essence of teamwork is learning how to bring out the best in one another.

T **10.** Maintaining emotional self-control is one way to demonstrate emotional intelligence.

STUDENT'S NAME   DATE   GRADE

HOW TO WIN FRIENDS AND INFLUENCE PEOPLE
By D. Carnegie
Galahad Books; New York, 1981

WHAT TO SAY WHEN YOU TALK TO YOURSELF
By S. Helmstetter
Grindle Press; Scottsdale, 1987

UNLIMITED POWER
By A. Robbins
Ballantine Books; New York, 1986

THE POWER OF POSITIVE THINKING
By N. V. Peale
Prentice Hall; Englewood Cliffs, NJ, 1978

senses

mirroring

communication

right-brained

appearance

stress

paraphrasing

Biological Powers

BIOLOGICAL POWERS

 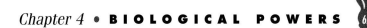

Perhaps you have heard the expression, "Beauty is in the eye of the beholder."

As beauty professionals it is important to recognize the biology behind the beauty.

The ability to see, smell, hear, taste and touch allows people to take in information from their surroundings. By appealing to clients' senses, successful stylists provide a pleasurable and stress-free salon experience.

This chapter describes how to take advantage of the senses in order to elevate clients' salon experiences. The relationship between mind, body and stress is also examined.

The key is discovering how to manage personal stress so that clients can relax and enjoy receiving their beauty services.

By the time you complete this chapter, you should be able to:
- Understand the importance of appealing to clients' senses.
- Use your senses to develop effective communication skills.
- Describe the difference between right- and left-brained individuals.
- Learn how to cope with personal stress.

Five Basic Senses

You might recall learning in elementary school that there are five basic senses. Each sense is controlled by a sense organ.

Sense: Sight
Sense Organ: Eyes

Sense: Smell
Sense Organ: Nose

Sense: Hearing
Sense Organ: Ears

Sense: Taste
Sense Organ: Mouth

Sense: Touch
Sense Organ: Nerve endings on the skin

The senses allow you to gather information from your surroundings. Imagine if you could not see, then you would be unable to drive. If you could not hear, then you would not be able to listen to your favorite CD. When using all five senses, you gain a more complete picture of your surroundings.

Successful stylists appeal to all of their clients' senses. Going to the salon should feel like spending time at a spa. This is a time for clients to escape daily hassles and stressful life experiences.

APPEALING TO THE SENSES

SENSE	STRATEGY	DIALOGUE
SEE	○ After styling, show clients their hair from different angles (front, side and back) by using mirrors. ○ Keep the salon immaculate. Make sure the bathroom is always clean and tidy. Make sure your station is clean.	*"Eighty percent of the time people are looking at you from an angle. Make sure you check your hairstyle from all angles."*
SMELL	○ Point out the pleasant fragrance of products that you use. ○ Before using a new product, ask the client if she likes the scent. ○ When using different products, make sure that the fragrances complement one another.	*"The minty scent of this shampoo will invigorate you and wake up your senses in the shower."*
HEAR	○ Play enjoyable music that appeals to a variety of ages and musical tastes.	*"Don't you love the beat of this music? It energizes me while I work."*
TASTE	○ Offer the client a drink or a snack.	*"Would you like something to drink while you relax under the dryer?"*
TOUCH	○ Pamper clients by giving them a scalp massage. ○ Help clients become familiar with their hair texture.	*"I want you to feel the dry ends of your hair. It could really benefit from a conditioning treatment."*

Focusing on Appearances ...

Beauty is often defined by appearance, so it is important to consider your own appearance and the appearance of your workstation. Check yourself frequently in front of the mirror to ensure you are presenting a professional image.

GENO SAYS:
"You are a walking advertisement for your own salon services."

DRESS

- Does my style of dress communicate professionalism?

- Are my work clothes appropriate for this salon?

- Are my shoes polished and clean?

GROOMING

- Am I practicing good grooming habits?

- How do I smell?

- What can I keep at work that will help maintain my appearance and hygiene?

POSTURE

- How do I carry myself when I walk and stand?

HAIR, SKIN & NAILS

- Does my hair look healthy and stylish?

- Is my skin healthy and vibrant?

- Do my nails look like they have just been manicured?

FACIAL EXPRESSIONS

- Is my smile pleasing to others?

- Do I make eye contact when others are talking to me?

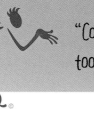

"Consider keeping the following items at work to refresh your appearance: toothbrush, toothpaste, mouthwash, deodorant and makeup."

The appearance of your workstation is just as important as your own appearance. When studying your workstation, imagine you are a client and look at the setting through the customer's eyes.

Analyzing the Workstation

SPACE

- Do work spaces meet minimum requirements?
- Can I service my client comfortably and safely?

SAFETY

- Have I followed the manufacturer's directions concerning my equipment's use and storage?
- Are my tools and station in good working order?
- Are there any spills on the floor or trip hazards that could cause my client injury?

CLEANLINESS

- Do I keep my work station clean and neat?
- Are my tools properly sanitized and labeled?
- Is the floor free of hair, dirt and water?

RA

Some regulatory agencies define minimum space requirements within salons. Check with the appropriate agency for requirements in your area.

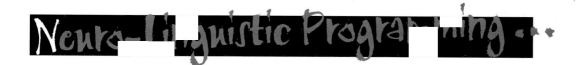

Using Your Senses to Communicate

As discussed in Chapter Two, communication is much more than just speaking. Effective communication includes verbal communication, nonverbal communication and active listening.

An exciting approach to communication called Neuro-linguistic programming (NLP) will help you connect with clients by focusing on their communication preferences. NLP is a method of communication that combines nonverbal behaviors and language. Mirroring and paraphrasing are two ways stylists use NLP to connect with clients and coworkers *(DuBrin, 2000)*.

HOW TO USE NLP...
MIRRORING

Mirroring happens when you imitate another person's physical behavior.

WAYS TO MIRROR OTHERS

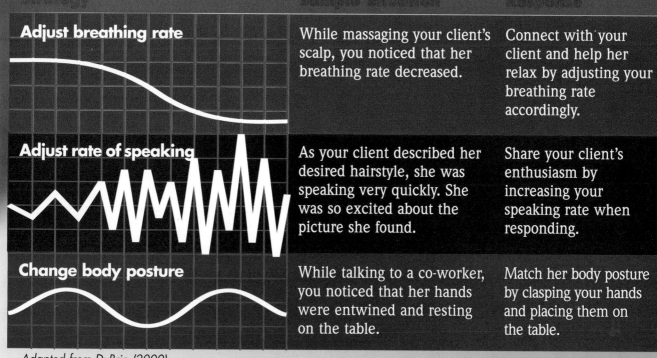

Strategy	Sample Situation	Response
Adjust breathing rate	While massaging your client's scalp, you noticed that her breathing rate decreased.	Connect with your client and help her relax by adjusting your breathing rate accordingly.
Adjust rate of speaking	As your client described her desired hairstyle, she was speaking very quickly. She was so excited about the picture she found.	Share your client's enthusiasm by increasing your speaking rate when responding.
Change body posture	While talking to a co-worker, you noticed that her hands were entwined and resting on the table.	Match her body posture by clasping your hands and placing them on the table.

Adapted from DuBrin (2000)

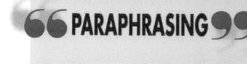

PARAPHRASING

Paraphrasing is another way to use NLP. As explained in Chapter Two, paraphrasing refers to using your own words to summarize what you heard the speaker say. When paraphrasing, focus on words that the client uses. If a client uses words that pertain to the senses, it provides clues about his or her mode of communication.

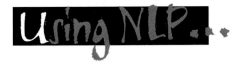

Three main modes of communication are: visual (eyes), auditory (ears) and kinesthetic (body) *(Robbins, 1986)*.

1 **Visual** communicators tend to focus on what they see. Paraphrase their statements and include phrases such as *"I see what you mean"* or *"It is clear to me."*

2 **Auditory** communicators listen and speak by relying mostly on their hearing. Capitalize on their mode of communication by using the phrase, *"It sounds like..."* or *"I hear you saying..."*

3 **Kinesthetic** refers to the body and its movements. Kinesthetic clients use their sense of touch to communicate. Paraphrase by using the words *"feel"* or *"felt."*

PARAPHRASE USING NLP

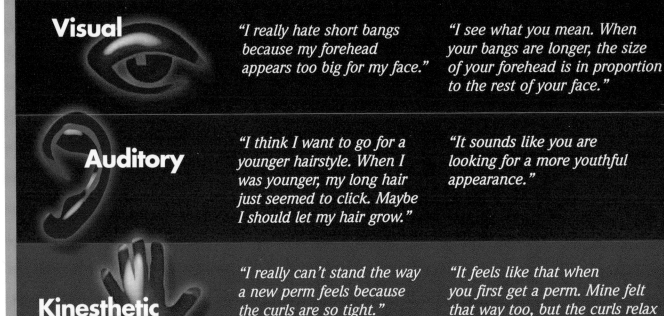

Communication Mode	Client Dialogue	Stylist Response
Visual	*"I really hate short bangs because my forehead appears too big for my face."*	*"I see what you mean. When your bangs are longer, the size of your forehead is in proportion to the rest of your face."*
Auditory	*"I think I want to go for a younger hairstyle. When I was younger, my long hair just seemed to click. Maybe I should let my hair grow."*	*"It sounds like you are looking for a more youthful appearance."*
Kinesthetic	*"I really can't stand the way a new perm feels because the curls are so tight."*	*"It feels like that when you first get a perm. Mine felt that way too, but the curls relax after about two weeks."*

Adapted from Robbins (1986)

As the preceding examples illustrate, studying the words that people use reveals interesting clues about their mode of communication. Some individuals rely more on their sense of sight to communicate whereas others rely on their sense of hearing or touch.

Besides communication preferences, people also differ with respect to their brain specializations. Significant research in this area came from studying patients whose brains had been split in half as a treatment for severe epileptic seizures *(Sperry, 1982)*.

During this radical "split-brain" surgery, fibers connecting both sides of the brain were severed. As a result, the two sides could no longer communicate. Studying "split-brain" patients provided doctors with important information about how the brain functions.

These interesting research findings have led communication experts to classify individuals as either right-brained or left-brained depending on which side is more dominant. When you identify your client's brain specializations, you'll be better able to explain beauty concepts and procedures to them.

Which Side of the Brain Does Your Client Favor?

(Edwards, 1999)

LEFT-BRAINED	RIGHT-BRAINED
Strengths: Verbal, analytical and logical abilities.	**Strengths:** Visual, spatial and creative abilities.
STYLIST APPROACH	**STYLIST APPROACH**
When Explaining Technical Information: Use specific words to describe the procedure and the end result.	**When Explaining Technical Information:** Provide a visual demonstration or show the client a picture.

1

"Adding this shade of highlights to your hair will add dimension, and will brighten your face."

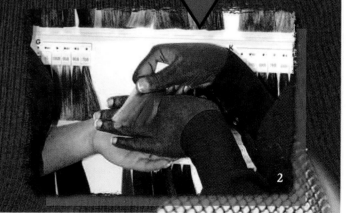

2

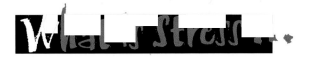

Stress is a perfect example of the mind-body connection because the way you think about life affects how your body feels. Stress is defined as physical and psychological responses to demanding situations. People often feel stressed when they interpret the demands of a situation as exceeding their resources for handling that situation *(Lazarus, 1999)*.

Stress can arise from both negative and positive situations. For example, stress is a common response after losing a job. Similarly, couples often feel stressed before their wedding day.

Whether stress stems from negative or positive factors, most people experience three phases of stress: alarm, resistance and exhaustion *(Selye, 1952)*.

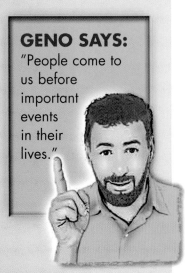

GENO SAYS:
"People come to us before important events in their lives."

Selye's Three Phases of Stress

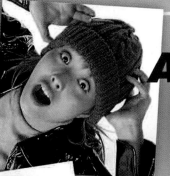

ALARM
The body becomes energized. The individual decides to either fight or flee.

RESISTANCE
The body adjusts to the threat by remaining in an anxious state. During this phase, individuals are susceptible to the negative effects of stress.

EXHAUSTION
The body cannot maintain a high state of readiness. Energy resources are consumed and the body starts to give up. Irreversible damage to the body is possible.

What Causes Stress ...

To effectively cope with stress, first identify the stressors in your life.

Factors that Cause STRESS

▶ **FEELING THAT YOU CANNOT CONTROL SPECIFIC FACTORS**

EXAMPLE: Lauren is in a traffic jam and feels stressed because she can't make the traffic move any faster.

▶ **TIME PRESSURES AND DEADLINES**

EXAMPLE: Brian is a stylist who feels stressed every time a beauty procedure takes longer than expected.

▶ **MOUNTING PROBLEMS**

EXAMPLE: Pauline has a habit of letting problems pile up until they reach a point where she feels overwhelmed.

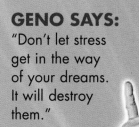

GENO SAYS:
"Don't let stress get in the way of your dreams. It will destroy them."

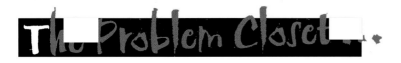

Stress is a common reaction when individuals ignore problems. Consider the following example of Jake and the problem closet.

Jake and the Problem Closet...

Jake is a young adult who does not like to deal with problems. He uses the problem closet in his mind to store them. He puts problems into the closet, closes the door and hopes they go away.

If a new stressor comes along, Jake thinks to himself, *"No worries, I'll just put it in the closet."* One day, Jake opened the closet and was bombarded by the problems that came tumbling out. Consequently, Jake's day was very stressful because he failed to realize there were so many problems in his life.

For two weeks, he worked on cleaning out the closet. The next time Jake encountered a problem, guess what he did? He put it in the closet and the problems began to pile up again.

FAMILY FINANCES JOB CAR

Coping with Stress

In order to avoid using the problem closet, ask yourself the following questions:

How can I solve the problem right now?

Is there someone who can help me solve it?

Is there some resource that I can use or study to help me solve it as soon as possible?

There are a variety of strategies for coping with stress. Consider trying the following approaches to find out which ones work best for you.

- Avoid procrastination.

- Engage in deep breathing exercises, meditation or yoga.

- Exercise.

- Talk about your problems with a friend or family member.

- Seek help from a professional counselor.

You can also try the following stress exercise to sort out the causes of your stress and decide whether or not you have control over the stressors.

STRESS EXERCISE

1. Draw a line down the middle of a piece of paper.

2. At the top write: "What I Can Control" on the left, and "What I Can't Control" on the right.

Think about the challenges in your life right now and decide on which list they belong.

4. Focus only on what you can control. Be willing to let go of what you cannot control.

What I Can Control . . .	What I Can't Control . . .
1.	1.
2.	2.
3.	3.
4.	4.
5.	5.
6.	6.

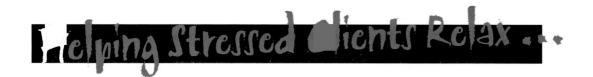

Beauty professionals frequently work with clients who are feeling stressed. A relaxed client will enjoy the salon experience much more than one who is stressed. Think about what you can do to make the salon experience more relaxing and enjoyable.

Stressed Client
Neisha is having her hair and makeup done before her engagement picture is taken.

Stylist Reaction
Recommend a cleansing facial using steamed towels and gentle exfoliation.

Stressed Client
Charlie is getting his hair colored before his high school reunion.

Stylist Reaction
Provide a scalp massage before the shampoo.

Stressed Client
Sandy is having her nails manicured before a job interview.

Stylist Reaction
Talk in a soft, calm voice as you instill confidence in Sandy.

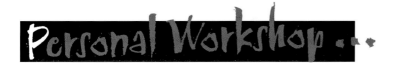
Personal Workshop...

Stress is an enemy when you let it get to you. Ask yourself the following reflection questions and use your responses to develop an Action Plan.

Reflection Questions

Stress Management Action Plan
I will...

Reflection Questions	Stress Management Action Plan — I will...
What causes stress in my life?	list all of the stressors in order from most stressful to least stressful.
Do I have control over these factors?	place each stressor into one of two columns (i.e., "What I Can Control" and "What I Can't Control"). be willing to let go of what I cannot control and focus only on what I can control.
Is there someone who can help me solve each problem?	record who can help solve the problem (e.g., friend, counselor, neighbor).
Is there some resource that I can use or study to help solve each problem?	identify the type of resource (e.g., book, item, website).
What can I do to manage my stress?	avoid procrastination. engage in deep breathing exercises, meditation or yoga. exercise.

On-line Resources

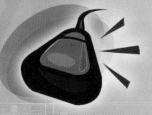

The internet provides access to a wealth of information about stress. The following websites pertain to stress and specific stress-related disorders.

Websites for Managing Stress

American Institute of Stress
http://www.stress.org

Medical Basis of Stress
http:/www.teachhealth.com

Medline Health Information
http://www.nlm.nih.gov/medlineplus/stress.html

American Psychological Association (APA)
http://www.apa.org/topics/topicstress.html

Diagnosing Stress
http://www.stressdiagnosis.com

Job-Related Stress
http://www.mindtools.com/smpage.html

Stress Management
http://www.stresstips.com

Screening Test for Depression
http://www.med.nyu.edu/psych/screens/odst.html

Anxiety Disorders
http://www.adaa.org

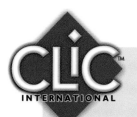

Biological Powers REVIEW QUESTIONS

MATCHING

___D___ **1.** A term used to describe someone who performs well on visual, spatial and creative tasks.

___E___ **2.** Physical and psychological responses to demanding situations.

___C / B___ **3.** Using your own words to summarize what you heard the speaker say.

___A___ **4.** A term used to describe someone who performs well on verbal, analytical and logical tasks.

___B / E___ **5.** Process by which the listener gives the speaker feedback about what was said.

A. Left-brained
B. Active Listening
C. Paraphrasing
D. Right-brained
E. Stress

TRUE OR FALSE

___F___ **1.** The phrase, *"It is clear to me,"* reveals a kinesthetic mode of communication.

___F___ **2.** The phrase, *"It sounds like,"* indicates an auditory mode of communication.

___F___ **3.** Right-brained individuals are smarter than left-brained individuals.

___F___ **4.** Stress only develops from negative situations.

___T___ **5.** The three phases of stress are: alarm, resistance and exhaustion.

___T___ **6.** Performing deep breathing exercises is one way to cope with stress.

___T___ **7.** Mirroring happens when you imitate another person's physical behavior.

___T___ **8.** Successful stylists appeal to all of their clients' senses.

___T___ **9.** Pointing out the pleasant fragrance of shampoo appeals to your client's sense of smell.

___T___ **10.** For right-brained clients, you should use pictures to explain technical information.

___F___ **11.** During the resistance phase of stress, the body becomes energized.

___T___ **12.** Avoiding procrastination helps to prevent stress.

___T___ **13.** You can mirror clients by adjusting your breathing rate to match theirs.

___T___ **14.** The senses allow you to gather information from your surroundings.

___T___ **15.** Analyzing the workstation means focusing on space, safety and cleanliness.

STUDENT'S NAME   DATE   GRADE

THE HEART AT WORK
By J. Canfield and J. Miller
McGraw Hill; New York, 1996.

DON'T SWEAT THE SMALL STUFF
By R. Carlson
Hyperion Books; New York, 1998.

THE ART OF HAPPINESS
By the Dalai Lama
Riverhead Books; New York, 1998.

STRESS WITHOUT DISTRESS
By H. Selye
Lippincott; Philadelphia, 1974.

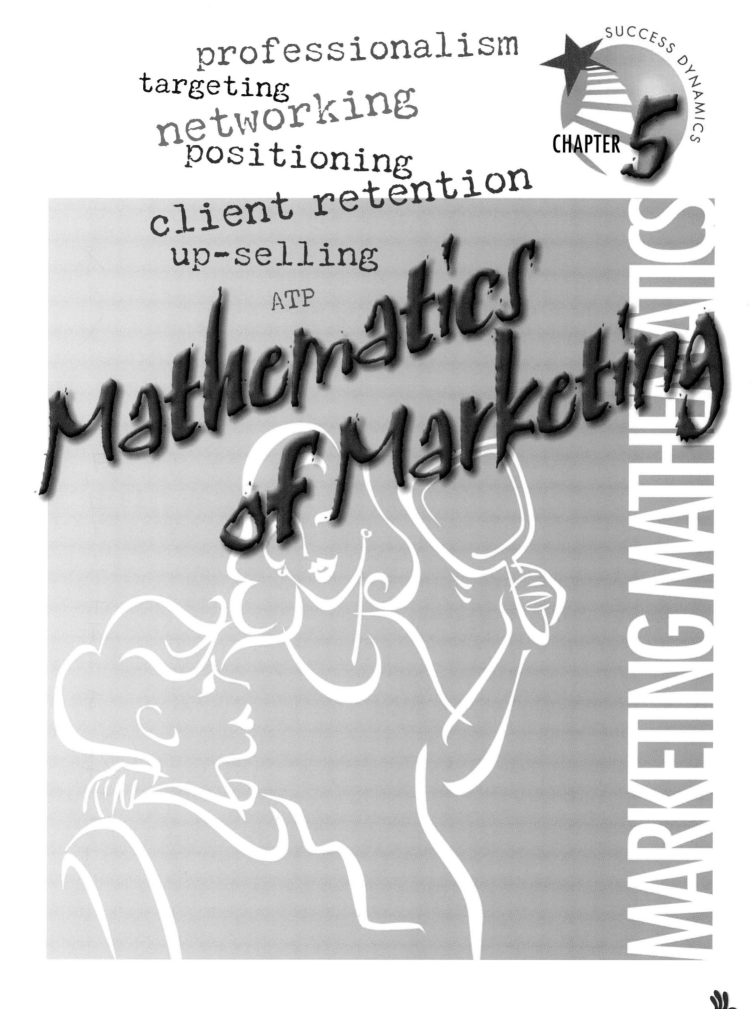

professionalism
targeting
networking
positioning
client retention
up-selling
ATP

Mathematics of Marketing

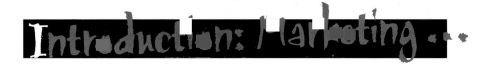

PERSONAL DEVELOPMENT

You are the president of your own Personal Development Company. As the president, you must strive to satisfy all of your clients. When clients are satisfied, they will continue to purchase beauty services and products from you. Understanding marketing is an important part of ensuring the success of your company. Marketing is the process of determining what customers need and then selling beauty services and products that satisfy those needs.

This chapter presents marketing strategies that will help you recruit new customers and retain existing ones.

Each person you come in contact with is a potential customer.

By the time you complete this chapter, you should be able to:
- Develop a comprehensive marketing plan.
- Utilize client retention strategies.
- Describe the marketing concepts of targeting, networking, recruiting and positioning.
- Know how to increase the average ticket price.
- Suggest ways to consistently satisfy customers and address their complaints.

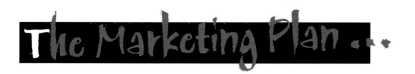

A comprehensive marketing plan is the key to success in the beauty industry. When developing the plan, ask yourself the following questions:

Are you
MEMORABLE?

The goal is to leave a lasting, positive impression on every person with whom you interact.

How do you
APPEAR
physically, mentally and emotionally?

Present yourself professionally and maintain a positive attitude.

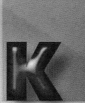

Are you
RESPONSIVE
to others' needs?

When meeting new clients, respond immediately by extending your hand to greet them. When responding to questions, lean forward and establish eye contact.

Do you **KEEP IN CONTACT** with people who are important to you?

Stay in touch with customers, friends and coworkers by keeping a current list of each group. Maintaining close relationships benefits both your personal and professional lives.

Do you
EVALUATE your plan of action?

Evaluate what you are doing to achieve your goals. Work smart. Just because you are working hard does not mean that you are working smart.

Are you
TARGETING
potential customers?

In the beauty industry, everyone is a target customer. Strive to meet three potential clients every day.

Professionalism...

A salon is a professional environment. Therefore, professionalism should be maintained at all times. Professionalism means behaving in a manner that is appropriate for a business setting.

Four Qualities of a Professional Stylist . . .

1
Avoid self-disclosure.
When conversing with clients, be careful not to disclose too much information about yourself. Refrain from discussing personal problems or issues in your life. Focus attention on your clients.

2
Always display a positive attitude.
If you are not feeling well, act as if you are feeling great. When you are unhappy, act as if you are happy.

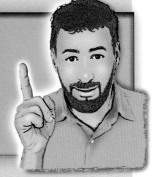

GENO SAYS:

"It is important to keep your personal life personal. Don't share information about yourself that will not benefit you."

3
Treat others with respect.
Always treat others the way you would like to be treated.

4
Be polite.
Say please and thank you, when speaking to clients and coworkers.

Building A Clientele ...

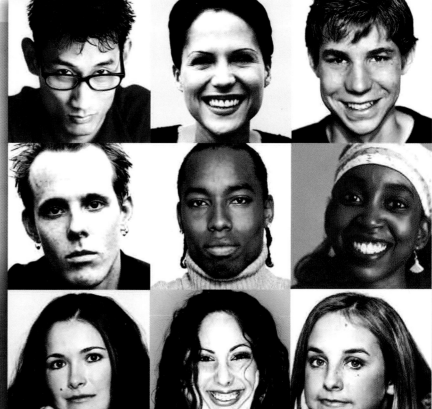

The cornerstone of success in the beauty industry is developing a loyal clientele.

This is the key to increasing revenue. Revenue refers to the money earned from the beauty services you provide.

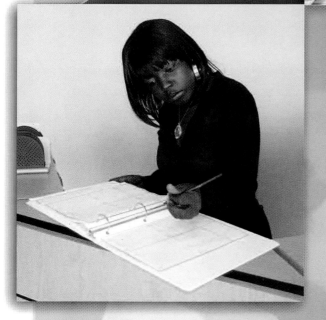

Four marketing principles will help you build a clientele:

○ **TARGETING**

○ **NETWORKING**

○ **RECRUITING**

○ **POSITIONING**

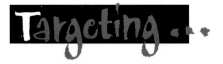

Directing marketing efforts toward those individuals who will most likely purchase your products/services is called targeting.

TARGETING

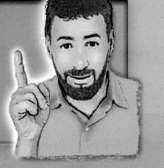

GENO SAYS:

"Every person you meet is a potential customer and a source of client referrals."

For most businesses, targeting involves considering a variety of consumer characteristics, such as geographic location, age and income level.

As beauty professionals, it is important to know who should be your target customers. The answer is simple – EVERYONE!

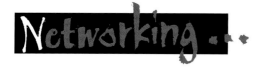

Networking...

Using social settings as an opportunity to meet potential customers is called networking. Each social group or event offers opportunities to expand your contacts. Use the four levels of marketing to increase your pool of potential clients.

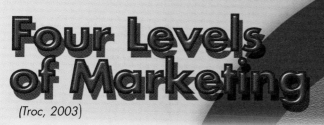

Four Levels of Marketing

(Troc, 2003)

CORE

Level One: The Core – Existing Customers
Develop your marketing plan by starting with the core. Then, work from the inside to the outer levels.

DIRECT CONTACTS

Level Two: Direct Core Contacts – Friends and Family
Ask for referrals. Satisfied clients are usually willing to refer their friends and family.

COMMUNITY MARKETING

Level Three: Community Marketing
Hand out business cards.
Compliment those around you.
Participate in children's organizations.
Be involved in community service organizations.

MASS MARKETING

Level Four: Mass Marketing
Advertise via newspapers, commercials, billboards and flyers.
For new businesses, awareness advertising lets potential customers know there is a new salon in town.

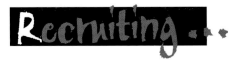

RECURITING

In the beauty industry, the primary source of new business comes from customer referrals. When choosing a stylist, people seek recommendations from trusted friends and family. The following strategies increase clients' willingness to provide referrals.

Client Referral Strategies

1 With every customer, use a personal script to request referrals.

"My greatest source of business is your personal referral. If you're pleased with our services, please tell your friends and family."

2 Implement a referral incentive program. Explain to clients that you will provide one free product or service for every new client they refer.

"Would you be interested in receiving free hair care for the rest of your life?"

3 Make sure every customer leaves with a few of your business cards. Distribute cards to any potential customer. Keep a supply at home, in your car and in the salon.

"Here are three business cards. Please give them to three people you know."

Positioning is the process by which clients develop positive associations about their stylist and the salon. By making each appointment a pleasant experience, customers develop positive mental images of you. As a result, you become the answer to your clients' beauty needs. What images do you want clients to have when calling to make appointments?

POSITIONING

My Stylist ...

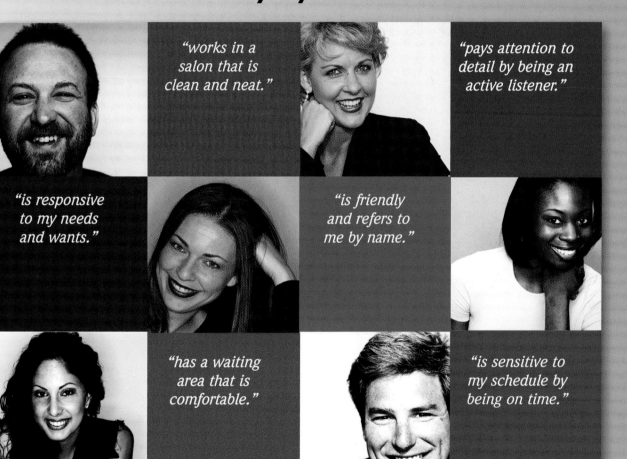

"works in a salon that is clean and neat."

"pays attention to detail by being an active listener."

"is responsive to my needs and wants."

"is friendly and refers to me by name."

"has a waiting area that is comfortable."

"is sensitive to my schedule by being on time."

"The salon is your stage and you are the star of the show. Make each performance award-winning, and your success will follow naturally."

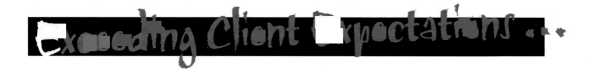

The key to a thriving business is exceeding customers' expectations. Added value is created when you give the customer more than was expected.

GENO SAYS:

"Promise less, but deliver more."

Formula for Exceeding Customer Expectations

What the Customer Received

—

What the Customer Expected

Added Value

How to Exceed Clients' Expectations

- Offer your client a beverage or a snack. People are more content when they are not hungry or thirsty.

- After a great manicure, walk the client outside, open her car door and start the engine.

- If it is raining, take an umbrella and walk your customer to her car.

Client Retention...

Keeping existing customers is called client retention. Follow these strategies to improve your retention rate:

Client Retention Strategies

1 Keep in touch with clients. Keep them informed of sales, new services and new products.

2 Send thank-you notes.

3 Call customers who have not been to the salon in a while.

4 Send holiday greeting cards to past and present clients.

5 Inform customers of special promotions via e-mail.

GENO SAYS:

"Develop life-long clients by giving added value to every client."

The following example demonstrates the power of client retention. During her first visit, customer Tracy and you talked about how highlights would greatly improve the texture and volume of her hair. Tracy agreed and scheduled her next appointment. For this first visit, Tracy's final bill was $40.25.

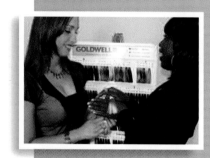

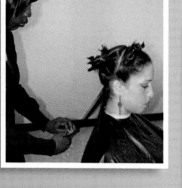

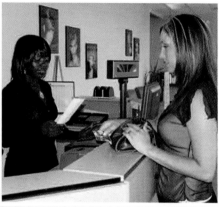

When Tracy returned to the salon six weeks later, you explained that using color–treated shampoo and conditioner prevents highlights from fading. As her second visit ended, Tracy purchased the recommended products. Her final bill was $122.75.

SECOND VISIT	
Haircut	$35.00
Highlights	$50.00
15% Tip	$12.75
Shampoo/Conditioner	$25.00
TOTAL:	**$122.75**

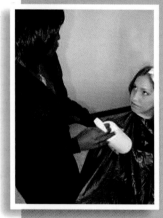

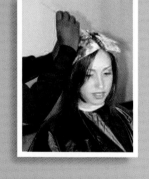

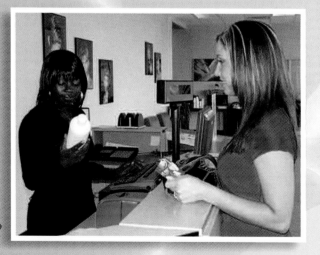

"Wow! Making one simple suggestion to Tracy more than doubled her service ticket. These are powerful techniques to master!"

Tracy is a conscientious client who wants her hair to look good all of the time. She returns to the salon every eight weeks for highlights. She continues to use the shampoo and conditioner that you recommend.

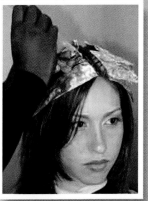

ANNUAL REVENUE

If Tracy re-books every eight weeks, you will see her at least six times a year:

TOTAL: $122.75 x 6 appointments = $736.50

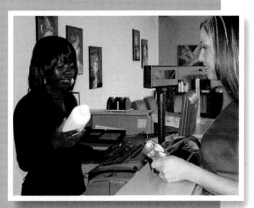

Tracy is so pleased with your beauty services and expertise that she refers her mother, best friend and coworker to you. These new customers also follow your advice and pay for an additional beauty service (e.g., perm, highlights or semi-permanent color). Now, the total revenue generated by retaining Tracy is almost three thousand dollars.

ANNUAL REVENUE

Tracy and three referred customers for one year:

Tracy	$736.50
Mom	$736.50
Best Friend	$736.50
Coworker	$736.50

TOTAL: $2,946.00

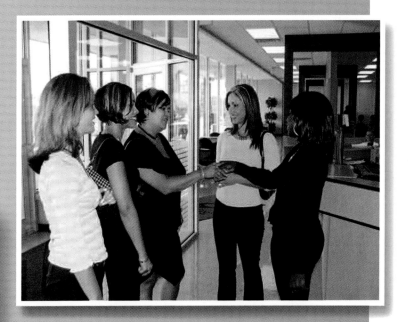

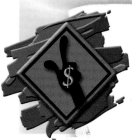

Combining the power of client retention with client referrals creates outstanding financial results.

Average Ticket Price...

Successful stylists constantly strive to increase the average ticket price (ATP) which directly improves their tips and commissions. The ATP is a formula for determining how much the typical client spends on services and products.

Calculating the ATP

Question	Answer
What were my total earnings today?	$300
How many clients did I serve today?	10
What is the average ticket price?	$30
($300/10 = $30.00)	

Increasing the ATP

Question	Answer
How can I increase the ATP by $10?	• Deep conditioning treatment
	• Clarifying treatment
	• Paraffin wax treatment for hands
	• Deep cleansing facial treatment
	• Small bottle of shampoo
How much will this increase my daily income?	$10 x 10 clients = $100
How much will this increase my weekly income?	$100 x 5 days = $500
How much will this increase my annual income?	$500 x 50 weeks = $25,000

Up-selling is increasing the amount of money each customer spends on beauty services and products. As shown in the example above, adding just ten dollars to every ticket increases your annual sales by twenty five thousand dollars!

GENO SAYS:

"Know what you have to sell and how much each service costs."

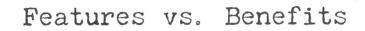
Successful salespeople get to know their customers and find out what is important to each one. When you know what your customers want, you will be more likely to sell services and products. First, know the features of each service and product, then tailor specific benefits to each client. A benefit for one client might be a disadvantage for someone else *(Ali, 2001)*.

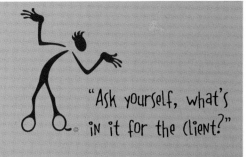

"Ask yourself, what's in it for the client?"

FEATURE=WHAT
BENEFIT=WHY

Focus on Features and Sell Benefits

Feature

Professional hair color...
provides long-lasting
color that does not fade.

Benefit

Client: Cash-strapped college student
"Professional products save money because the color lasts longer than store-bought products."

A perm...
is trendy, minimizes frizz
and provides extra fullness.

Client: Working mother who has little free time
"A perm will shorten your morning routine by at least 15 minutes and your hair will look great all of the time."

Acrylic nails...
are resistant to chips
and breakage.

Client: Jewelry Designer
"Having beautiful acrylic nails will help you sell more jewelry."

This method is applied when you present the customer with a small, initial suggestion. This suggestion, in turn, increases the chance that the customer will later agree to a larger suggestion. Research indicates that this is an effective selling strategy *(Cialdini, 1993)*.

Consider the following example. Your goal is to increase revenue by selling to an existing customer named Joanne. During the consultation, you suggest that adding a few highlights could add brightness and dimension to Joanne's hair. Joanne seems a little hesitant because she has never used color before. So, you recommend adding just a few highlights around her face for ten dollars. Joanne agrees and is very satisfied with the results. In fact, Joanne is so pleased that she schedules another appointment for all-over highlights.

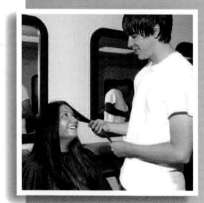

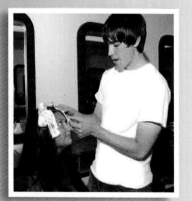

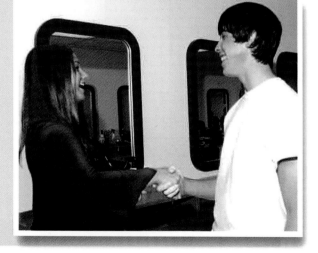

Sales Strategies ・・ Value vs. Price

Successful selling

involves imagery. The goal is to create pictures in customers' minds that make the value of the service or product worth more than the price.

Most customers are willing to pay more for quality professional beauty products. When customers are unhappy with their beauty products, they typically discontinue using them. For example, Marquita purchased a bottle of conditioner at the drug store for five dollars. Whenever she used this product, her hair remained dry and frizzy. So, Marquita threw away the new conditioner. In other words, she wasted the money used to purchase this unsatisfactory product.

"Store-bought products end up costing more when they fail to deliver satisfactory results."

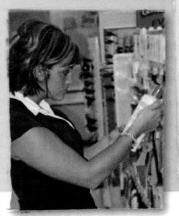

Customer satisfaction is a critical component of client retention. Use a personal script to ensure that every customer who leaves the salon is satisfied with your beauty services.

"Have you ever returned a meal to a restaurant's kitchen because you were completely dissatisfied with it? Did they replace it? If so, you'll probably go there again."

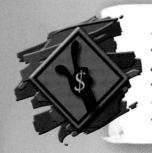

IF EVER SOMETHING SHOULD HAPPEN HERE THAT WOULD PREVENT YOU FROM COMING BACK, PLEASE LET ME KNOW.

The Guarantee

Providing a money-back guarantee helps to ensure customer satisfaction. Clients feel more trusting of their stylist when products and services are guaranteed. If a client knows that she can return a product for a full refund, she will be more willing to try it. The same principle applies to guaranteed beauty services. Customers' willingness to take risks and try new services increases when you provide free follow-up appointments if they are dissatisfied with the services received.

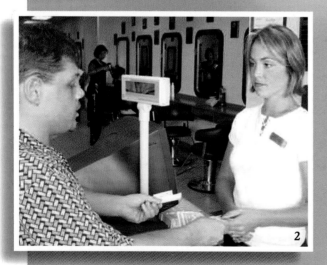

Professionals view complaints as an opportunity for business growth. Always listen intently and do whatever it takes to make sure your customers are satisfied and delighted.

Customer Complaints...

Client complaints are an inevitable part of working in the beauty industry. There are two goals when working with client complaints:

1 Minimize the number of complaints.

2 Bring every complaint to a successful resolution that is fair to both client and stylist.

"Sometimes, it may be necessary to interrupt a dissatisfied client. For instance, if she is speaking in a loud voice, ask her to speak quietly inside the salon."

Before responding to complaints, make sure you understand why the client is upset. If a client seems reluctant to state her concern, try one of the following phrases:
"Tell me what happened," or *"Tell me why you are upset."*
While the client expresses her complaint, use active listening, but avoid interrupting her.

most of the time

AVOID INTERRUPTING

ACTIVE LISTENING

The following steps provide a framework for addressing client complaints immediately and appropriately:

Responding to Client Complaints *(Dubrin, 2000)*

Strategy	Script
1 Acknowledge the client's point of view, but avoid placing blame.	*"You're upset because ..."*
2 Apologize for the error.	*"I'm sorry that this happened."*
3 Enlist the client as a partner.	*"Let's work together to see how we can solve this problem."*

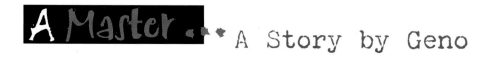

The greatest form of marketing is to be a master at what you do. When considering examples of great service, take note of a master. A master comes in all different forms. Who would ever think that you could find a master hot dog vendor? Consider the following true story from co-author Geno Stampora.

MARKETING

THE MASTER HOT DOG VENDOR

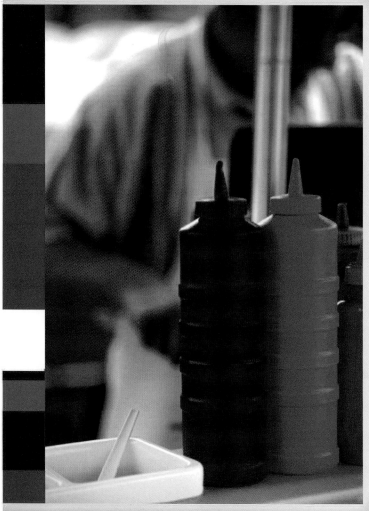

"I was speaking to a group of beauty professionals at the Cleveland Convention Center. At lunchtime, I was interested in finding a quick lunch so I walked outside and looked at all of the hot dog vendors. In the distance, I spotted a hot dog stand with a new, colorful umbrella.

As I approached the stand, the older fellow greeted me in a raspy, but friendly voice. He made eye contact and said, *'I'm so glad that you chose my stand. You look like a two-hot-dog gentleman.'* Before I could respond, he continued, *'I could give you one now and hold the other one to keep it hot.'* The vendor then asked, *'What is your choice of drink?',* and pointed to five drinks on the shelf. He kept it simple by only having five drinks to choose from. In a matter of seconds, I had purchased two hot dogs and a soda.

I took my first bite and said, *'Your hot dogs are delicious.'* The man replied, *'The most important thing in my business is to have delicious hot dogs and a clean, brightly colored umbrella.'* He continued, *'My umbrella is my marketing tool, which is why I replace it every six months.'*

This man was a master hot dog vendor. He prepared his script, used great eye contact and knew the importance of an effective marketing tool."

Personal Workshop ...

Successful marketing efforts are only possible when you are content with your personal and professional lives. Life-enriching experiences are all around you. Ask yourself the following reflection questions and use your responses to develop an Action Plan.

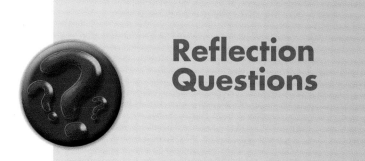

Reflection Questions

Personal Growth Action Plan

I will ...

How can I enrich my life?

visit museums and study beautiful works of art.

appreciate nature.

read inspiring biographies.

surround myself with positive people.

How can I make my career more rewarding?

continuously review my short-term, intermediate and long-term goals.

monitor my progress.

celebrate each success.

What can I do outside of work that will enhance my career?

be involved in my community.

join local professional organizations.

What strategies comprise my marketing plan?

develop an unforgettable method of telling, showing and sharing with others what I do.

While working, how can I put myself in a position of positive focus at all times?

act as a magnet by pulling the best of others toward me.

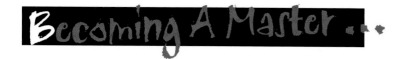

Think for a moment about the incredibly talented athletes whose goal it is to win a medal at the Olympics. These athletes undergo years of relentless training and practice in order to increase their odds of achieving the ultimate goal – a gold medal.

While preparing for the big event, athletes rely on the wisdom, knowledge, and experience of their coaches. After closely monitoring and observing practice sessions, coaches predict which refinements will lead to a successful outcome. This valuable feedback enables athletes to make improvements that increase their odds of achieving victory. Becoming a master in the beauty industry also requires a constant pursuit of knowledge, guidance and new experiences. With CLiC as your coach, you are on your way!

MATCHING

G **1.** Behaving in a manner appropriate for a business setting.

A **2.** Process by which the listener gives the speaker feedback about what was said.

E **3.** Utilizing social settings as an opportunity to meet new clients.

H **4.** Money earned from the services provided.

J **5.** Process by which stylists determine what customers want and then sell beauty services and products that satisfy their clients' needs.

I **6.** Directing marketing efforts toward those individuals who are identified as most likely to purchase the service/product.

C **7.** Keeping existing clients.

F **8.** Process by which clients develop positive associations about the stylist and the salon.

D **9.** Increasing the amount of money each customer spends on beauty services and products.

B **10.** A formula for determining how much the typical client spends on beauty services and products.

A. Active Listening

B. Average Ticket Price (ATP)

C. Client Retention

D. Marketing

E. Networking

F. Positioning

G. Professionalism

H. Revenue

I. Targeting

J. Up-selling

TRUE OR FALSE

F **1.** The formula for exceeding client expectations is supply minus demand.

T **2.** Every person you meet is a potential client.

F **3.** Superb technical skill is the most important part of selling beauty services and products.

T **4.** The foot-in-the-door technique increases the likelihood that a customer will comply with you request to purchase beauty services/products.

F **5.** Clients are generally more trusting of stylists who offer a money-back guarantee.

F **6.** When responding to client complaints, you should never apologize for your mistake.

T **7.** Referral incentives increase clients' willingness to recommend your services to others.

T **8.** The four levels of marketing are core, direct contacts, community marketing and mass marketing.

F **9.** In the beauty industry, the primary source of new business comes from targeting adolescents.

T **10.** Your personal problems should not be discussed with clients.

STUDENT'S NAME   DATE   GRADE

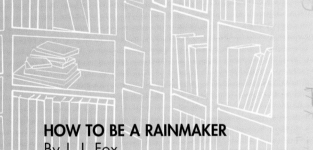

HOW TO BE A RAINMAKER
By J. J. Fox
Hyperion Publishing; New York, 2000.

WHAT IT TAKES TO BE #1
By V. Lombardi
Mc-Graw Hill; New York, 2001.

MARKETING WARFARE
By J. Trout and A. Reis
McGraw Hill; New York,1986.

SEE YOU AT THE TOP
By Z. Ziglar
Pelican Publishing; Gretna, LA, 1975.

dialogue

impression management

rapport   closed question

consultation

finishing

revenue

The Art of Service Delivery

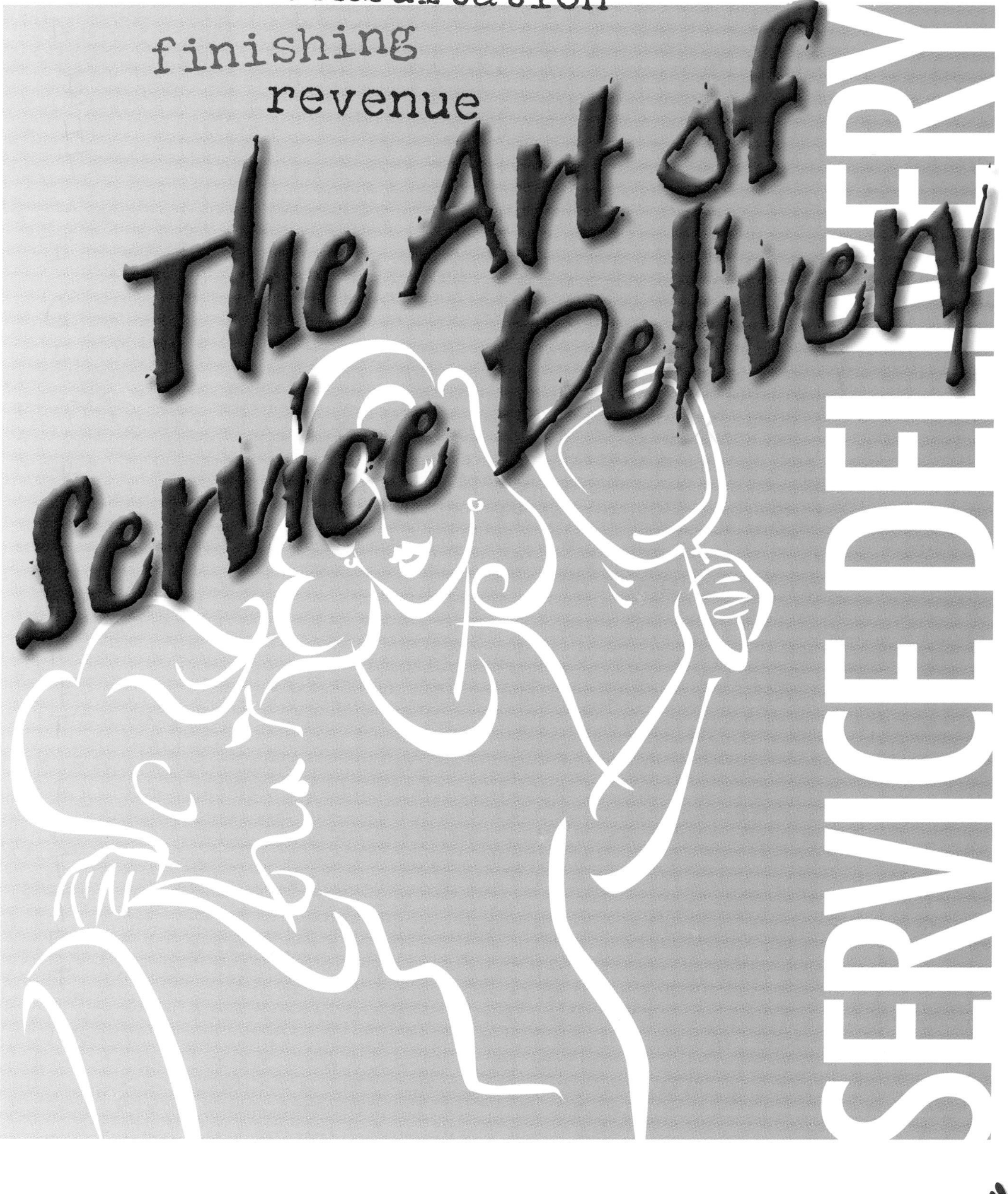

SERVICE DELIVERY

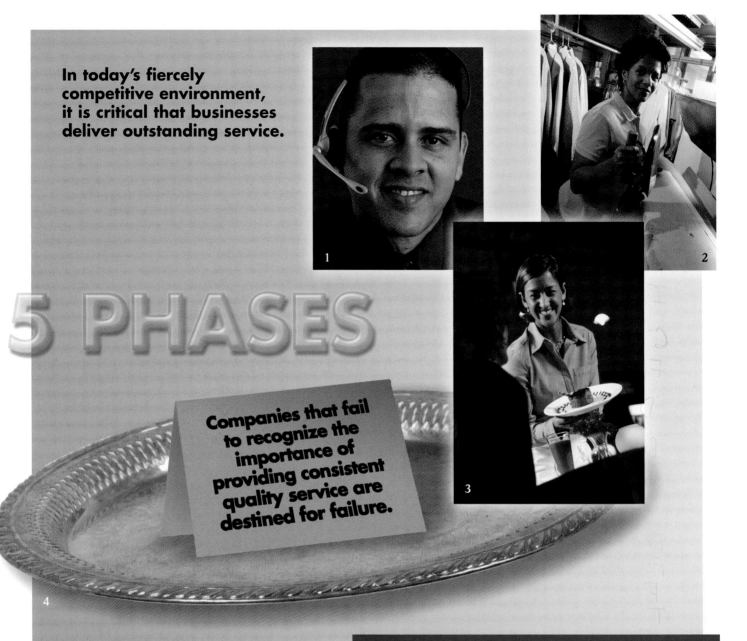

In today's fiercely competitive environment, it is critical that businesses deliver outstanding service.

5 PHASES

Companies that fail to recognize the importance of providing consistent quality service are destined for failure.

1

2

3

4

This chapter provides a description of the service delivery process. By building on previous concepts, the chapter explains how to deliver first-rate service by incorporating communication skills, people skills and marketing strategies.

By the time you complete this chapter, you should be able to:

- Learn how to recognize and provide great service.

- Describe the five phases of service delivery.

- Understand the importance of first impressions.

- Know how to use self-enhancing strategies.

- Improve your conversation skills.

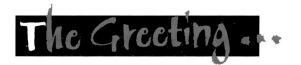

1 APPROACH THE CLIENT

2 MAKE EYE CONTACT

3 EXTEND YOUR RIGHT HAND FOR A HANDSHAKE

4 USE YOUR GREETING SCRIPT

Phase 2

This phase begins when the client enters the salon. The greeting is more than just saying hello to clients. It incudes introducing yourself, giving a positive impression and making an initial connection.

To greet clients use the following four steps: approach the client, make eye contact, shake hands and use your greeting script.

Acknowledge clients within 10 to 15 seconds. Try using a smile, wave or eye contact initially. Later, approach the client and extend your hand.

Even though there is a sense of familiarity with repeat clients, always offer a professional greeting coupled with a handshake.

GREET

GREETING SCRIPT

For New Clients:
"Hi, Miles. It is very nice to meet you. My name is Sarah. I am excited about working with you today. Let's talk for a few minutes before we get started."

For Repeat Clients:
"Hi Miles. It is nice to see you again. I am excited about working with you today. Let's talk about what you would like to accomplish today."

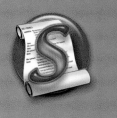

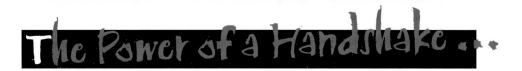

The handshake is the most widely accepted introduction in a business relationship for both men and women. Before shaking someone's hand, first try waiting for the client to stand. If the client remains sitting, be aware of what might be placed on her lap that could interfere with the handshake (e.g., purse, drink, or magazine).

"Always be considerate of your clients' time, schedule and feelings."

Making the Handshake

Once the client is standing, establish eye contact and offer a friendly smile. Lean forward and be the one who takes the other's hand. Aim for the full hand shake.

The handshake should be firm, but sensitive. Make your grip strong and positive.

Be sure not to use too much force. The handshake should not create discomfort.

Avoid the "dead fish" handshake, which is characterized by a very loose grasp.

Impression Management

As the old saying goes, you never get a second chance to make a good first impression. First impressions are critical in the beauty industry. Your livelihood depends upon how others view you. Most clients will not return to someone they do not like.

Impression management refers to attempts to control how others perceive you. Use self-enhancing strategies to create positive first impressions. Self-enhancing strategies improve the way you appear to others *(Seta, Paulus & Baron, 2000)*.

"The more attractive you are to yourself, the more attractive you'll be to others."

Stand tall and speak with confidence.

Self-Enhancing Strategies

Look in the mirror and ask yourself, "Do I look like a beauty professional?"

DRESS FOR SUCCESS

Your style of dress is a powerful communication tool. Be careful about displaying tattoos and body piercings when trying to build business in mainstream society. For example, if you wear a nose ring, it is unlikely that the mother of a nine-year-old will bring her daughter to you for a haircut for fear that her daughter might want a nose ring too.

PERSONAL GROOMING

Remember that you are working within the client's personal bubble. Avoid too much perfume or cologne. Wear clothes that are freshly laundered. Make sure that you have fresh breath. Avoid gum chewing and smoking.

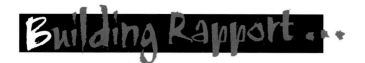
Building Rapport...

When you first get to know clients and develop a close connection with them, it is called rapport. Establishing rapport helps the client feel comfortable communicating with you.

Strategies for Building Rapport with Clients

DISPLAY A POSITIVE ATTITUDE
Clients prefer to spend time with people who have a positive outlook on life.

BE WARM AND INVITING
Think of clients as guests who have come to visit in your home. Be hospitable to clients and welcome them into the salon.

USE EFFECTIVE COMMUNICATION TOOLS
Utilize verbal and nonverbal communication strategies that convey you are interested in learning more about your client.

BE UPLIFTING
Successful stylists leave clients feeling better about themselves and their lives.

BE A CREDIBLE BEAUTY EXPERT
Your clients are paying you to make them look their best. Gain clients' trust.

After establishing rapport, you earn the right to proceed to the next phase, which is the consultation.

"The key to establishing rapport is building comfort and instilling confidence in the customer's mind."

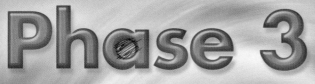

Consultation...

Obtaining information from the client in order to provide excellent service is called **consultation**. The beginning of the consultation process can be described as "information-in" because you take in as much information as possible about the client's hair, skin, or nails. During this phase, **active listening** is critical to ensuring customer satisfaction.

Phase 3

During the consultation, communication breakdowns can be prevented by using **paraphrasing** and visual communication. Visual communication helps to clarify the client's message by relying on signs, symbols and objects to communicate.

Examples of Visual Communication

Justin requests that the stylist trim one inch off the back of his hair. The stylist asks Justin to use his fingers and show how much is an inch.

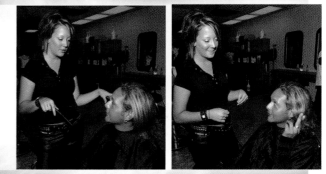

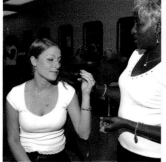
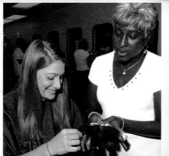

Barbara asks her stylist to dye her hair strawberry blonde. The stylist refers to color swatches so that Barbara can choose the exact shade of strawberry blonde.

CONSULT

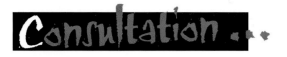

Consultation...

QUESTION

Asking appropriate questions is critical to the consultation process. As discussed in Chapter 2, open questions usually begin with "How," "What," or "Why." Closed questions, in comparison, usually begin with "Is," "Are," or "Do." Consultation scripts vary depending on the type of service. Here are some sample questions that can be used to determine what the customer wants to accomplish.

INFORMATION-IN

HAIR	NAILS	SKIN
• *What do you love about your hair?*	○ *Do your nails flake periodically?*	• *How would you describe your skin type?*
• *Is there anything that you don't like about your hair that you would like me to correct for you?*	○ *Is chipping or cracking a problem?*	• *Where are your trouble spots?*
	○ *What is your desired nail length?*	• *Have you noticed that your skin's needs change with the seasons?*
• *If you could do anything at all with your hair, what would that be?*	○ *What is your ideal nail shape?*	• *Are you satisfied with the tone and color of your skin?*
		• *What is your skin care regimen?*

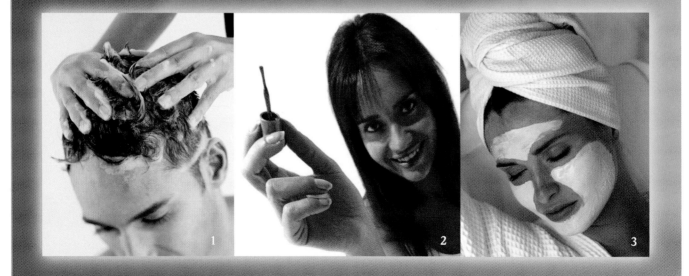

Use the following strategies to prevent miscommunication during the consultation process.

STRATEGY	DIALOGUE
Ask follow-up questions to determine whether the client was satisfied with the previous service.	*"Tell me how you feel about the haircolor that we used last time."*
Use open questions rather than closed questions.	*"What do you have in mind for today?"* *"What can I do for you today?"*
Use paraphrasing to ensure clear communication.	*"You think that longer hair would make you look more youthful."* *"I see what you mean. When your bangs are longer, the size of your forehead is in proportion to the rest of your face."*
Clarify unclear statements to avoid miscommunication.	***Client:*** *"My hair is just a mess. You know what I mean. My hair is one of my biggest problems."* ***Stylist:*** *"I really want to make sure I understand. Tell me specifically what you don't like about your hair."* *OR . . .* ***Client:*** *"I can't stand my hair. It's too big! "* ***Stylist:*** *"Tell me what you mean when you say your hair is 'too big'."*

The information-in process comes to life when delivering services. Based on information shared during the consultation, you perform the requested service. The service may be applying acrylic nails, giving the client a facial or a perm.

Phase 4

DELIVER

Service is the longest phase of the process. It encompasses the following components:

1 Preparing for the service.

2 Delivering great service.

3 Selling additional services and products.

4 Conversing with clients.

Preparing for the Service

Service preparation depends on the type of service being performed.

Service Examples

Type of Service:
Makeup Application
Preparation:
Remove existing makeup and cleanse the face and neck.

Type of Service:
Manicure
Preparation:
Remove old polish and soak the hands.

Type of Service:
Haircut
Preparation:
Shampoo and condition hair.

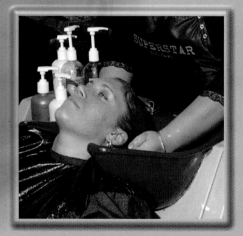

Part of preparing for the service is explaining what you are about to do. For instance, before shampooing, put the product in your hand and show the client what you are going to use on her hair.

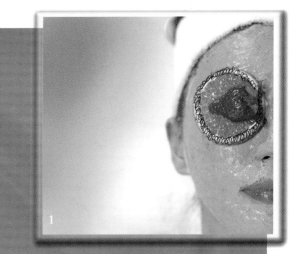

Making sure your clients' needs are met is essential to ensuring customer satisfaction and client retention. As discussed in Chapter Five, successful stylists take specific steps to consistently exceed clients' expectations. Additional recommendations are provided below.

SERVICE DELIVERY IN THE SALON

PAMPER CLIENTS
Make sure clients are comfortable. The salon environment should be relaxing and pleasing to the eye.

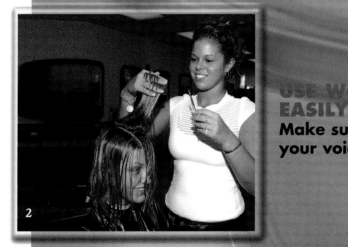

USE WORDS THAT ARE EASILY UNDERSTOOD
Make sure that sincerity can be heard in your voice as you explain procedures.

SERVICE

OFFER YOUR PROFESSIONAL BEAUTY RECOMMENDATIONS
Recommend specific services and products that will improve your client's hair, skin and nails.

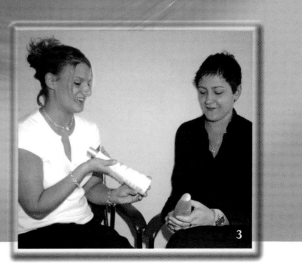

"Talk business while working on your clients."

As described in Chapter Five, up-selling is the key to increasing revenue. Use the following strategies to increase the ticket price:

SUCCESSFUL APPROACHES TO UP-SELLING

Strategy	Description	Dialogue
Educate clients about the services and products that are available.	Describe specific features of these services and products and how they will benefit the client.	*"Today, I'm going to use a shampoo designed specifically for curly hair. This product gives definition to curls and combats the effects of humidity."*
Interest the customer in additional services and products.	Use words that produce vivid pictures in the customer's mind.	*"Highlights give dimension, thickness, texture, shine and depth to your hair."*
Showcase professional products.	Help clients understand the many benefits of professional products.	*"Professional products will last longer than store-bought products because they are more concentrated."*
Plant the seed for additional services.	Suggest specific ways the client can improve the appearance of her hair, skin, or nails.	**Hair** *"As I'm cutting your hair, I'm thinking about how great it would be to add some highlights. Let's do a test strand to give you an idea of how it would look."* **Skin** *"While cleansing your skin, I noticed some fine lines. I can remove most of them with a series of microdermabrasion treatments. I'll give you some information about the process when I show you the skincare products."* **Nails** *"Our salon has many services and products that will improve the strength of your nails. Why don't we set aside some time next week to try a fiber wrap?"*

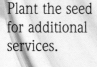

Providing opportunities for clients to purchase professional products leads to increased revenue and client retention.

Client Preferences for Conversation

TYPE	EXPLANATION	STYLIST RESPONSE

ALL BEAUTY — Client wants to have long discussions about her hair, skin or nails. — Talk about the client's beauty attributes. Focus on her thick wavy hair or her flawless skin. Provide lengthy, detailed explanations about the services you are providing.

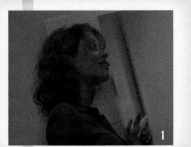

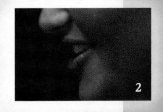

While providing great service, focus all of your attention on the client. Do not take phone calls or initiate conversations with anyone else. Give clients the opportunity to control conversation topics.

Although no two conversations are the same, most clients can be categorized into three general types with respect to their conversation preferences.

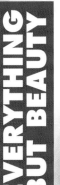

EVERYTHING BUT BEAUTY — Client wants to talk about herself or be entertained by stimulating conversation. — Follow the client's lead. If she wants to talk, use active listening. If she wants to be entertained, talk about what is happening in the news or in the entertainment industry. Tell a humorous story.

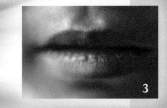

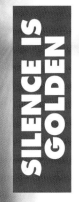

SILENCE IS GOLDEN — Client wants to relax and be pampered. She does not want to be bombarded with an endless number of questions. — Temporary silence is the best approach. Wait for the client to initiate conversation. Concentrate on your work and help the client relax. Savor the silence.

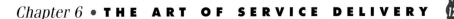

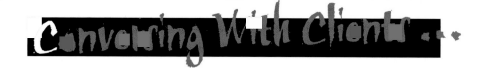

Being a professional stylist is an occupation where conversing with others is a critical part of providing service. Successful stylists strive to be great conversationalists.

A Great Conversationalist...

- always has interesting topics to discuss.
- talks about current events.
- can engage anyone in "small talk."
- uses nonverbal and verbal encouragers.

Encourage clients to continue talking by nodding your head in agreement, displaying a facial expression that reflects interest or concern and using encouragers, such as "hmm" or "uh-huh."

A great conversationalist will always be worth more to clients than a top-notch stylist who has poor communication skills.

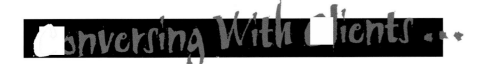

Conversing With Clients ...

Clients decide how great your technical service is by how well you communicate with them.

Use the following eight strategies to improve your conversation skills:

1
Ask about clients' families and friends by name. This shows that you are interested in learning more about the important people in their lives.

2
Remember important facts about your clients' lives. (e.g., sick aunt, stressful job, helpful daughter-in-law) Jot this information down on the client record card after each service.

3
Talk business while working with clients. Focus on their hair, skin and nails.

4
Tailor the topic of conversation to fit each client's interests, background and experiences (e.g., hobbies, travel, and occupation). Avoid too much self-disclosure.

5
Address the client by name during the conversation (e.g., *"Sharon, I couldn't agree more."*).

6
Always have a variety of back-up topics (e.g., movies, books, TV shows, local news and weather).

7
Keep your conversations confidential. Avoid gossiping about clients or coworkers.

8
Avoid topics that might insult or offend clients. For instance, never discuss sex, drugs, politics, religion or any other topic that could develop into a negative conversation.

"The way you talk about others tells clients how you are going to talk about them after they leave."

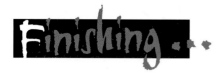

FINISH
Phase 5

The last phase of the service delivery model is finishing. This phase starts with putting on the final touches and ends when the client leaves the salon. This is the most important phase of the service delivery process, yet it is often neglected or overlooked completely.

Strive to deliver the final phase in a way that will make you stand out against the competition. Ask yourself, "What can I do that will make my clients tell their friends and family about what a great beauty professional I am?"

For stylists, putting on the finishing touches is like telling the world, "Hey, look at my masterpiece." This phase is similar to the final step a gourmet chef takes when garnishing a dessert.

Show clients how to do their hair. Remember that you are the expert. Give them confidence by saying,

"You can do this at home. I will show you how."

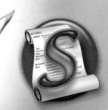

Home Maintenance Personal Prescription
FOR_____
STYLIST_____
SHAMPOO_____
CONDITIONER_____
STYLING AIDS_____
FINISHING PRODUCT_____

FINISHING STRATEGIES

- Give clients a home maintenance prescription for their hair, including the appropriate tools and products.

- Before you close, show clients the finished product. For example, ask clients to hold a hand-held mirror while you show them the back of their hair.

- Showcase and sell the tools that you use. Emphasize the importance of using proper tools.

GENO SAYS:
"While many stylists lose their steam during the finish, the true professional gains momentum."

Final Closing Steps . . .

Many beauty professionals are not with their clients when it is time for them to leave. Some people think that they are too busy to close with clients, however, this step is far too important to overlook. It is the best time to market additional services and products.

STEP 1 — WALK THE CLIENT TO THE RECEPTION AREA

Walk beside the client and stay on the same side of the desk. Your job is to make clients look and feel their best. Whenever possible, let the receptionist take the client's money.

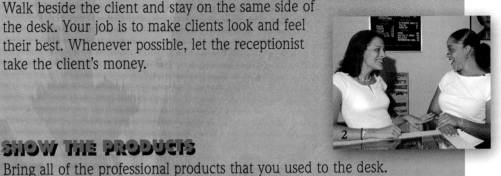

STEP 2 — SHOW THE PRODUCTS

Bring all of the professional products that you used to the desk.

CLOSING PRODUCT SCRIPT

"These are all of the products that I used and this is what I recommend that you take home."

Record the recommended products and note which were purchased. During the next appointment, ask follow-up questions to determine if the client was satisfied with the purchased products.

STEP 3 — BOOK THE NEXT APPOINTMENT

If your salon works by appointment, then book the next appointment before the customer leaves.

RE-BOOK SCRIPT

"The most important part of my job is making sure that your hair always looks its best. I recommend that you book your next appointment for 6-8 weeks from now."

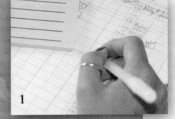

STEP 4 — EXPRESS YOUR GRATITUDE

THANK YOU SCRIPT

"Thank you so much for your business. It was a pleasure spending time with you. I look forward to seeing you again."

Scripts •• Quick Reference Guide

The words you use are important to your business success. Scripted dialogue is essential for excellent service delivery. Get comfortable by practicing with others.

Professionals with a marketing strategy and dialogue skills positively influence clients' purchasing decisions.

Using Different Types of Scripts

ACT 1:
SCENE 1:

CONSULTATION

Purpose: Assure clients that your goal is to satisfy their requests and exceed their expectations.

Consultation Script: *"Kim, in order to be sure that we are on the same page, I'd like you to describe your beauty routine."*

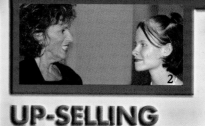
2

GREETING

Purpose: Make a lasting, positive impression.

Greeting Script: *"Hi, Amanda. It is very nice to meet you. My name is Steve. I am excited about working with you today. Let's talk for a few minutes before we get started."*

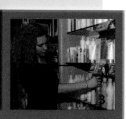

UP-SELLING

Purpose: Establish your expert status by sharing your knowledge of hair, skin and nails. Plant the seed.

Up-Selling Script: *"As I'm cutting your hair, I'm thinking about some ideas for color that would really enhance your skin tone and eye color."*

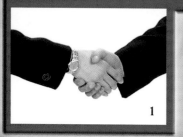
1

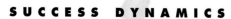

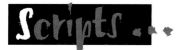

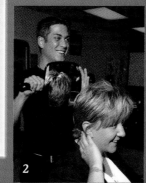

FINISHING

Purpose: Educate clients so that they can follow the beauty routine at home. Instill confidence.

Finishing Script: *"You can do this at home. I'll show you how."*

CLOSING

Purpose: Make your professional recommendations.

Closing Script: *"These are the products that I used and this is what I recommend that you purchase."*

Purpose: Schedule the next appointment.

Re-Book Script: *"The most important part of my job is making sure that your hair always looks its best. I recommend that you schedule your next appointment for 6-8 weeks from now."*

Purpose: Express gratitude.

Thank you Script: *"Thank you very much for your business. It was a pleasure spending time with you. I look forward to seeing you again."*

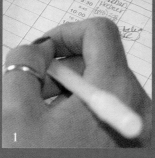

PREVENTING CLIENT COMPLAINTS

Purpose: Make sure that every customer is a fan.

Complaint Script: *"My greatest source of business is your personal referral. If you're pleased with our services, tell your friends and family. If not, let me know and I will fix the problem."*

ADDRESSING CLIENT COMPLAINTS

Purpose: Ensure that every customer is satisfied.

Complaint Script: *"I'm sorry that this happened. Let's work together to see how we can solve this problem."*

NETWORKING

Purpose: Use a non-stop marketing campaign to build business.

Networking Script: *"I work at an innovative salon only 20 minutes from here. We offer the full range of services. Here's my card. I hope to see you in the salon soon."*

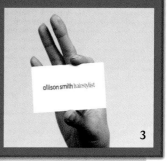

allison smith hairstylist

Learn how to provide excellent service by finding great service examples and studying them. Then, think about how those examples can be incorporated into your business. Ask yourself the following reflection questions and use your responses to develop an Action Plan.

Reflection Questions

Service Action Plan

I will ...

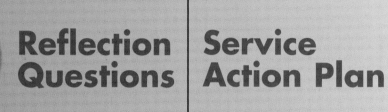

Who are the masters that I know?

identify at least three different masters.

_____

_____

_____

What are the qualities of great service?

determine specific indicators of excellent service delivery.

_____

_____

How can I incorporate those qualities into my business?

describe ways that I can incorporate these indicators into my own business.

_____

_____

_____

_____

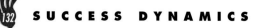

MATCHING

B 1. Question that can be answered in a few words.

E 2. Attempts to control how others perceive you.

A 3. Using your own words to summarize what you heard the speaker say.

C 4. Obtaining the information you need from the client in order to provide excellent service.

D 5. Last phase of the service delivery model which begins with putting on the final touches and ends when the client leaves the salon.

F 6. A question that invites the receiver to provide additional information.

J 7. Increasing the amount of money each customer spends on beauty services and products.

I 8. Money earned from the services provided.

G 9. Process by which the receiver gives the speaker feedback about what was said.

H 10. Developing a close connection with someone you meet.

A. Active listening
B. Closed question
C. Consultation
D. Finishing
E. Impression management
F. Open question
G. Paraphrasing
H. Rapport
I. Revenue
J. Up-selling

TRUE OR FALSE

F 1. Greeting is the first phase of the service delivery model.

F 2. Successful stylists do not talk very much.

F 3. You should only shake clients' hands when you meet them for the first time.

T 4. Consultation is described as the "information-in" phase.

F 5. An example of visual communication is asking the client to show you how long she wants her nails sculpted.

F 6. If "Silence is Golden" describes your client's preference for conversation, you should introduce many different topics of conversation.

T 7. Addressing the client by name is an effective conversation strategy.

T 8. The final step in the finishing phase is scheduling the next appointment.

T 9. To establish rapport, stylists should tell clients all about themselves.

F 10. Masters are people who completed high school.

STUDENT'S NAME   DATE   GRADE

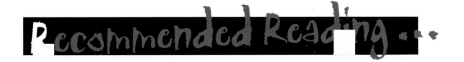

DISCOVERING THE SOUL OF SERVICE
By L. L. Berry
Simon & Shuster; New York, 1999

RAVING FANS
By K. Blanchard
William Morrow & Co.; New York, 1993

LEADERSHIP IS AN ART
By M. De Pree
Bantam Doubleday; New York, 1989

SELF MADE IN AMERICA
By J. McCormack
Addison Wesley; New York, 1990

POUR YOUR HEART INTO IT
By H. Schultz
Hyperion Publishing; New York, 1997

active listening
client retention
jargon
personality
rapport
consultation
assertiveness

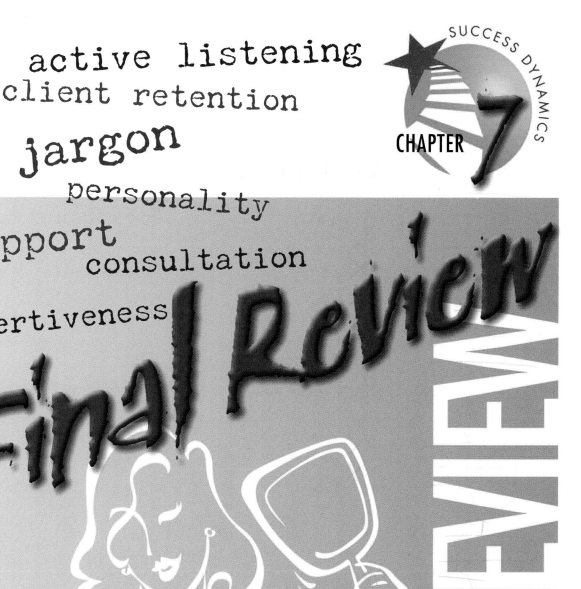

Final Review

FINAL REVIEW

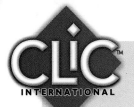

Success Dynamics FINAL REVIEW QUESTIONS

FILL-IN-THE-BLANK

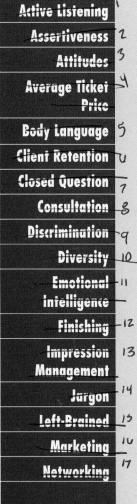

Active Listening — 1
Assertiveness — 2
Attitudes — 3
Average Ticket Price — 4
Body Language — 5
Client Retention — 6
Closed Question — 7
Consultation — 8
Discrimination — 9
Diversity — 10
Emotional Intelligence — 11
Finishing — 12
Impression Management — 13
Jargon — 14
Left-Brained — 15
Marketing — 16
Networking — 17

1. _Closed question_ is a question that can be answered in a few words.

2. _Jargon_ refers to words or phrases that only beauty professionals know.

3. _Assertiveness_ is an honest, open expression of one's thoughts and feelings.

4. _Client Retention_ is keeping existing clients.

5. _Body Language_ refers to communication cues provided by the movement and position of your body.

6. _Active Listening_ is the process by which the listener gives the speaker feedback about what was said.

7. _Discrimination_ is unfair behavior directed toward members of another group.

8. Your evaluation of the world around you is called _Attitudes_.

9. A term used to describe someone who performs well on verbal, analytical and logical tasks is _left brained_.

10. Utilizing social settings as an opportunity to meet new clients is called _Networking_.

11. _Consultation_ refers to obtaining the information you need from the client in order to provide excellent service.

12. The last phase of the service delivery model which begins with putting on the final touches and ends when the client leaves the salon is called _Finishing_.

13. _Average ticket price_ is a formula for determining how much the typical client spends on beauty services and products.

14. _Diversity_ refers to distinct differences between people.

15. Attempts to control how others perceive you is called _Impression Management_

16. _Marketing_ is the process of determining what customers need and then selling beauty services and products that satisfy those needs.

17. The ability to monitor your own and others' feelings and use this information to guide behavior is called _Emotional Intelligence_

STUDENT'S NAME   DATE   GRADE

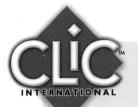
FILL-IN-THE-BLANK

Nonverbal Communication
Open Question
Paraphrasing
Personality
Personality Trait
Positioning
Prejudice
Professionalism
Rapport
Revenue
Right-Brained
Self-Actualization
Self-Esteem
Slang
Stereotype
Stress
Targeting
Up-Selling

18. Developing a close connection with someone you meet is called ___Rapport___.

19. ___open question___ is a question that invites the receiver to provide additional information.

20. ___Slang___ refers to informal words which are typically inappropriate for professionals to use.

21. Behaving in a manner appropriate for business setting is called ___Proffesionalism___

22. ___Self-Esteem___ is an unspoken language consisting of eye contact, facial expressions, and body language. ___non-verbal Communication___

23. ___Self-esteem___ refers to an overall evaluation of your self-worth.

24. ___Stereotype___ is a widely held belief about people who share a common trait or belong to a particular group.

25. ___Personality___ is an individual's unique combination of psychological characteristics and behavior patterns.

26. An unfair or negative attitude about another group is ___prejudice___.

27. Behavioral descriptor that explains the way people are in most situations is called ___Personality trait___.

28. The term used to describe someone who performs well on visual, spatial, and artistic tasks is ___Right-Brained___.

29. ___Up-Selling___ is increasing the amount of money each customer spends on services and products.

30. The need to develop to your fullest potential is called ___Self-actualization___.

31. ___Paraphrasing___ is using your own words to summarize what you heard the speaker say.

32. ___Revenue___ refers to money earned from the services provided.

33. ___targeting___ refers to directing marketing efforts toward those individuals who are most likely to purchase the service or product.

34. ___positioning___ refers to the process by which clients develop positive associations about their stylist and the salon.

35. ___Stress___ refers to physical and psychological responses to demanding situations.

STUDENT'S NAME   DATE   GRADE

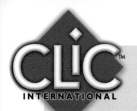
TRUE OR FALSE

_T_ **1.** Individuals with the Type A personality are competitive.

_T_ **2.** Offering an apology helps to resolve conflicts.

_T_ **3.** Assertive beauty professionals speak with confidence.

_F_ **4.** Conflicts are an inevitable part of life.

_T_ **5.** Sitting with your arms folded across your chest suggests unhappiness.

_F_ **6.** Open questions can be answered in a few words.

_T_ **7.** Attitudes may be positive, negative or neutral.

_F_ **8.** Compared to individuals with high self-esteem, individuals with low self-esteem are more motivated and productive at work.

_T_ **9.** For some people, low self-esteem comes from a personal belief that they are not smart.

_T_ **10.** Paraphrasing helps to prevent communication problems.

_T_ **11.** Characteristics of an effective voice include using inflections.

_T_ **12.** Nonverbal communication is more difficult to control than verbal communication.

_F_ **13.** Direct eye contact is socially appropriate in all cultures.

_F_ **14.** Joining community organizations is an example of mass marketing.

_T_ **15.** Sitting slumped in a chair could suggest shyness.

_T_ **16.** Assertive people respectfully express their opinions.

_F_ **17.** People who are extroverted are shy and reserved.

_F_ **18.** Conscientious clients are usually late for appointments.

_T_ **19.** Agreeable clients are understanding if you are running behind schedule.

_T_ **20.** Exercise is a strategy for coping with stress.

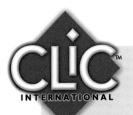

MULTIPLE CHOICE

1. Empathetic responses are used to:
   A. understand your point of view.
   B. show you understand someone else's thoughts/feelings.
   C. provide a summary of the points made by someone else.
   D. establish yourself as an expert.

2. What is the final step in the finishing phase?
   A. Walking your client to the reception area
   B. Showing the products that you used
   C. Scheduling the next appointment
   D. Thanking your client

3. Which of the following is an open question?
   A. *"Do you want something to drink?"*
   B. *"Is the water temperature too hot?"*
   C. *"Are you going to get a manicure?"*
   D. *"What is your skin care regimen?"*

4. Which of the following is NOT one of the goals of communication?
   A. To express
   B. To understand
   C. To facilitate understanding
   D. All of the above are goals of communication.

5. Slang refers to using:
   A. words of acceptance, such as *"I see"* and *"Okay."*
   B. informal words such as *"ain't."*
   C. words that only beauty professionals know.
   D. assertiveness skills.

6. What of the following is NOT one of the three main types of communication?
   A. Active listening
   B. Verbal communication
   C. Assertiveness
   D. Nonverbal communication

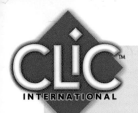

MULTIPLE CHOICE

7. Which type of communication relies on body language to send messages?

   A. Verbal communication

   B. Nonverbal communication

   C. Active listening

   D. None of the above

8. Paraphrasing is using your:

   A. ears to take in information.

   B. own words to summarize what was said.

   C. expertise to persuade the client.

   D. eyes to read the client's thoughts and feelings.

9. Paraphrasing is important because it shows the speaker that you:

   A. heard what was said.

   B. are a beauty expert.

   C. use words of acceptance.

   D. understand the rules of proximity.

10. Which of the following statements includes jargon?

   A. *"My Momma told me that I should open my own beauty shop."*

   B. *"I'm gonna add some volume to your hair by using this round brush."*

   C. *"If you look in this mirror, you'll be able to see the back of your hair."*

   D. *"Your hair is very porous."*

11. An effective strategy for resolving conflicts is:

   A. blaming others.

   B. raising your voice.

   C. addressing the conflict directly.

   D. avoiding people.

12. Which of the following behaviors conveys a positive attitude?

   A. Criticizing

   B. Lying

   C. Complaining

   D. Offering praise

STUDENT'S NAME   DATE   GRADE

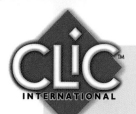
MULTIPLE CHOICE

13. People who have high self-esteem view their own failure as providing:
    A. client referrals.
    B. important feedback about how to improve.
    C. negative information.
    D. insulting information.

14. Which of the following is NOT one of the Big Five Traits?
    A. Conscientiousness
    B. Extroversion
    C. Agreeableness
    D. Compassion

15. Nonverbal communication includes which of the following components?
    A. Body language
    B. Facial expressions
    C. Eye contact
    D. All of the above

16. Which of the following is NOT one of the keys to high self-esteem?
    A. Set reasonable, but challenging goals.
    B. Realistically take credit for your successes.
    C. Recognize when failure occurs due to factors outside of you.
    D. All of the above are keys to high self-esteem.

17. A characteristic of the Type B personality is:
    A. repeatedly looking at your watch.
    B. fidgeting in your seat.
    C. speaking quickly.
    D. speaking in a soft, calm voice.

18. Which of the following strategies is recommended when working with "know-it-all" clients?
    A. Use empathetic statements.
    B. Use open-ended questions to encourage them to talk.
    C. Ask for their opinion and advice.
    D. None of the above

STUDENT'S NAME   DATE   GRADE

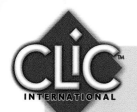

Success Dynamics FINAL REVIEW QUESTIONS

MULTIPLE CHOICE

19. Which of the following is an example of discrimination?

    A. Refusing to hire a stylist because of her age

    B. Refusing to give a haircut to a client in a wheelchair

    C. Both A and B are examples of discrimination.

    D. Neither A nor B is an example of discrimination.

20. Selye's three phases of stress are:

    A. alarm, resistance and exhaustion.

    B. auditory, visual and kinesthetic.

    C. concern, cooperation and respect.

    D. exercise, meditation and counseling.

21. Which of the following is a client retention strategy?

    A. Keeping in contact with clients by sending thank you notes

    B. Calling clients who you have not seen in a while

    C. E-mailing clients to inform them of sales and other promotions

    D. All of the above

22. Which of the following is an example of a personal script to request referrals?

    A. *"My greatest source of business is your personal referral. If you like what you see, please tell your friends and family."*

    B. *"Here are three business cards. You must know three people you can send me."*

    C. Both A and B are correct.

    D. Neither A nor B is correct.

23. Which stylist is using the "foot-in-the-door" technique?

    A. Jim talks to his client about the benefits of using professional products.

    B. Mary first suggests adding a few highlights before recommending all-over highlights for her client.

    C. Rachel recommends cutting her client's hair before applying a conditioning treatment.

    D. As soon as the client enters the salon, Mario explains the foiling process to her.

24. Goals of addressing client complaints include:

    A. bringing every client complaint to a successful resolution.

    B. minimizing the number of client complaints.

    C. Both A and B are correct.

    D. Neither A nor B is correct.

STUDENT'S NAME   DATE   GRADE

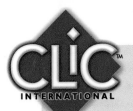
MULTIPLE CHOICE

25. When addressing client complaints, you should:

A. blame someone else for the problem.

B. ignore the client.

C. respond by saying, *"I'll try harder next time."*

D. apologize for the error.

26. Which of the following scripts applies to enlisting the customer as your partner?

A. *"Let's work together to see how we can solve this problem."*

B. *"You think that shorter hair looks better on you."*

C. *"I really couldn't say whether a perm would be a good look for you."*

D. *"I found that this product works very well on oily hair."*

27. Which of the following invites the listener to share more information?

A. *"Guess what I did last night."*

B. *"I am really tired today."*

C. *"Tell me more about it."*

D. *"Yesterday, I gave my first perm."*

28. Suzie is a new client. You notice that she is constantly rubbing her hands together while she sits in the chair. Based on body language cues, it is likely that Suzie is:

A. angry.

B. nervous.

C. disappointed.

D. lazy.

29. Personal bubble refers to the:

A. boundary of intimate space.

B. use of non-verbal encouragers.

C. degree of hair volume.

D. need for self-esteem.

30. A universally recognized gesture that communicates happiness is:

A. frowning.

B. yelling.

C. smiling.

D. yawning.

STUDENT'S NAME   DATE   GRADE

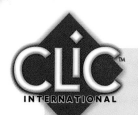
BEHAVIOR EVALUATION

Use your best judgment to rate the following behaviors as professional or unprofessional.
Describe each statement using the following key:
P = Professional
U = Unprofessional

1. __U__ Chewing gum while performing a manicure.

2. __U__ Looking down at the floor while talking to your client.

3. __U__ Telling your client how unhappy you are with your present boyfriend.

4. __U__ Asking your client about his political affiliation.

5. __U__ Asking your client to explain why she divorced her husband.

6. __U__ Telling the receptionist that you are having a bad day because you are hung over.

7. __P__ Giving business cards to potential clients.

8. __U__ Being rude to a coworker because you think she "stole" your client.

9. __P__ Using social functions as an opportunity to grow your business.

10. __U__ Taking a phone call in the middle of giving your client a facial.

11. __U__ Counting your tips while standing at your station during business hours.

12. __P__ Smiling and thanking your client for her business at the end of the service.

13. __U__ Wearing torn blue jeans and dirty shoes at work.

14. __U__ Sharing personal client information with a coworker.

15. __P__ Writing the name of purchased products on the client's record card.

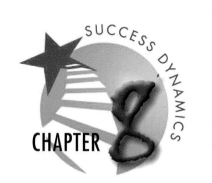

success

time management

road map

goal setting

interview

resume

portfolio

Extra Credit

EXTRA CREDIT

SUCCESS DYNAMICS

CHAPTER 8

 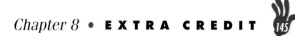

SUCCESS

Beauty school is a time
to develop skills and
practice strategies that
will lead to your success.
Seeking feedback and input
from other beauty professionals
will sharpen your skills.
Do not let any minor detours
end your drive toward success.
Instead, let them serve as a
powerful motivating force
to help you overcome
temporary roadblocks
on the journey to success.

This chapter explains how to take a proactive role when planning for success by creating a road map, interviewing beauty professionals, developing a resume, and participating in a mock interview.

By the time you complete this chapter, you should be able to:
- Learn how to manage time more effectively.
- Identify your short-term, mid-range, and long-term goals.
- Develop a goals sheet.
- Identify the skills necessary for landing your first job.
- Improve your resume and portfolio.

Fundamentals of Selling...

Achieving success in any aspect of life requires the ability to sell. Sales efforts are a major part of our relationships, personal happiness, and life successes. Great salespeople understand how to showcase themselves and their services.

The two major keys to selling are knowledge and understanding. You must know your craft and the tools you use. Practice talking about the services and products that you offer.

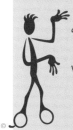

"Always have faith and confidence in who you are and what you do."

UNDERSTANDING

SALES

KNOWLEDGE

Time Management ...

There never seems to be enough time.
Successful people learn how to use time in the most productive ways. They learn how to accomplish more and more in one day. If you put value on a minute, you will not want to waste it.

Below are some key ideas for time management:

Do

- Get organized in every aspect of your life.
- Set priorities and follow them.
- Create a time list for the day.

Don't

- Waste others' time.
- Squander time.
- Be late for appointments and meetings.

GENO SAYS:
"Make every moment matter and you will master time."

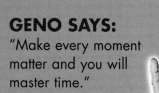

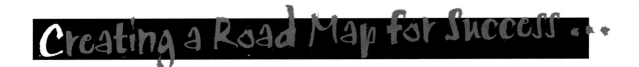

Creating a Road Map for Success ...

Just like driving directions tell travelers how to get from one city to the next, road maps for success provide beauty professionals with the path to realizing their goals.

The greatest benefit of having a road map is that you have an inner-persistence and motivation for life that many people never acquire. People who have a road map also develop an inner voice that says, *"I will do whatever it takes to achieve my goals."* This inner voice produces the energy needed to achieve long-term goals because you are constantly inspiring yourself and experiencing short-term gratification. Creating a road map starts with personal goal setting.

GENO SAYS:
"Without setting goals for your life and career, you'll never reach your full potential."

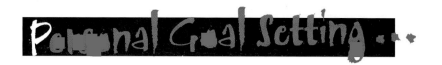

GENO SAYS:
"What you focus on is what gets done."

Personal goal setting begins with understanding your mission and how important goals are to achieving success. Unfortunately, for many people goal setting is a negative experience because they set goals and then fail to achieve them. Often this happens when goals are either unrealistic or unachievable within the specified time frame.

Road maps for success include three types of goals: short-term, mid-range and long-term.

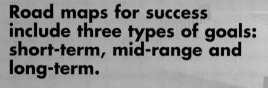

3 TYPES OF GOALS

Type	Duration	Purpose
Short-Term	One day to one month	• Keep you on track. • Provide momentum.
Mid-Range	One month to one year	• Create a sense of accomplishment. • Build discipline.
Long-Term	One year to end of life	• Serve as the ultimate reward; the pot of gold at the end of the rainbow.

Personal Goal Setting...

In determining what your goals should be, begin by asking yourself specific questions:

Goal Setting Questions

Defining Goals

- What do I want to be?
- Where do I want to go in life?
- What is my desired income level?
- How long do I want it to take to fill my "book"?
- Is my goal achievable?

Creating a Road Map

- What are the things that I need to do, read, or research in order to make this goal a reality?
- Who can help me achieve this goal? (e.g., who are my resources?)
- How will I measure my progress?

SHORT-TERM duration=1mo.	MID-RANGE duration= 1 yr.	LONG-TERM duration=10 yrs.
By the end of one month, I will sell professional products to 35% of my clients.	By the end of one year, I will be the number one retailer in my salon.	Within ten years, I will own my own salon.
I will save 10% of my daily income every day for a month.	By the end of the year, I will develop the additional income to complete payment on my student loans.	In ten years, I will save #130,000. toward retirement.
I will find 12 new clients that I will be excited to work with by the end of the month.	I will develop 130 new clients a year.	In ten years, I will choose my clientele, so I do not have to work with walk-ins.

Stay on track by reviewing your goals often.

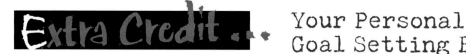

The goal setting process can be broken down into three practical applications.

1 Interview three beauty service professionals.

2 Ask three salon owners to evaluate your resume and portfolio.

3 Participate in a mock job interview with a salon owner.

1. INTERVIEW BEAUTY PROFESSIONALS

Develop ten interview questions that will help you identify the qualities of successful beauty professionals. Using these ten questions, conduct three interviews with beauty professionals in your area. Look for the concepts that have been addressed throughout the book. Consider the following areas: communication skills, personality traits, marketing strategies, conversing with clients, and service delivery.

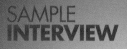

SAMPLE INTERVIEW

1. What strategies do you use when marketing services and products to clients?

2. How do you recruit new clients?

3. What are the keys to client retention?

4. How do you handle client complaints?

5. What do you do to exceed your clients' expectations?

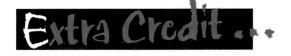

Extra Credit...

2. RESUME AND PORTFOLIO REVIEW

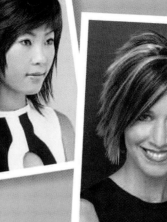

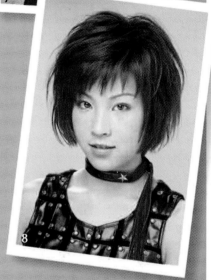

The resume is a communication tool that summarizes your education, employment history and professional accomplishments. When a resume is coupled with a professional portfolio, it increases your chances of finding employment. A professional portfolio showcases your skills and abilities by providing actual illustrations and examples of your beauty expertise.

After developing your resume and professional portfolio, share it with three salon owners and ask for their feedback.

"The feedback samples on this page may be used as a guide for collecting feedback."

SAMPLE
RESUME FEEDBACK

1. Is the resume well organized?

2. Does it provide sufficient information?

3. Does it contain the information you look for when selecting potential employees?

4. How can it be improved?

SAMPLE
PORTFOLIO REVIEW

1. Does the portfolio showcase excellent technical skills?

2. Is the portfolio comprehensive?

3. How can it be improved?

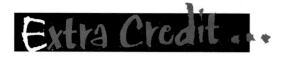

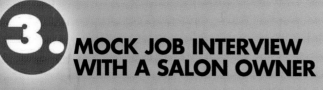

First, schedule a meeting with a salon owner and ask the owner to evaluate your interviewing skills.

After the interview is completed, write a one-page reflection paper analyzing your interview. Write about what you would do differently during the next interview.

"A sample cover letter and interview evaluation form are included to assist you with this exercise."

SAMPLE COVER LETTER

Date

Dear Salon Owner,

_____ would like to begin by thanking you for
(Beauty School Name)

your participation in the mock interview process. For purposes of

this exercise, please regard the student as a potential candidate

for employment.

Use the attached rating scale to evaluate this potential candidate on

a scale of 1 to 5. A score of 5 means that the candidate displayed strong

hiring potential in this area. A score of 1 means that the individual did

not demonstrate the attributes/skills necessary for employment in this

area. In addition, any comments you have are greatly appreciated.

If you have any questions, please contact me at _____.
(Beauty School Phone Number)

Sincerely,

_____
(Beauty School Instructor)

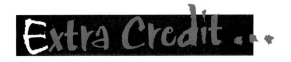
HAIR
SKIN
NAILS

MAKE-UP

CONFIDENCE

GREETING

Rating Scale for Mock Interview

1=LOW 5=HIGH

INTRODUCTION

Areas to consider:
handshake, eye contact, greeting

1 2 3 4 5

PROFESSIONAL APPEARANCE

Areas to consider:
clothes, hair, make-up

1 2 3 4 5

KNOWLEDGE

Areas to consider:
hair, skin, nails

1 2 3 4 5

BEHAVIOR

Areas to consider:
confidence, energy level,
willingness to adhere to your
salon's standards

1 2 3 4 5

INTERPERSONAL SKILLS

Areas to consider:
communication skills
posture, eye contact

1 2 3 4 5

COMMENTS

_____
_____
_____
_____

References ...

Ali, M. (2001). *Marketing effectively.* London: Dorling Kindersley.

Baron, R. A., & Byrne, D. (2002). *Social psychology* (10th ed.). Boston: Allyn & Bacon.

Bramson, R. M. (1997). *Coping with difficult people.* New York: Ballantine.

Brophy, J. (1998). *Motivating students to learn.* Boston: McGraw Hill.

Coon, D. (2003). *Essentials of psychology* (9th ed.). Belmont, CA: Wadsworth/Thomson Learning.

Costa, P. J., Jr., & McCrae, R. R. (1987). Personality in adulthood: A six-year longitudinal study of self-reports and spouse ratings on the NEO personality inventory. *Journal of Personality & Social Psychology, 54,* 853-863.

DePaulo, B. M. (1992). Nonverbal behavior and self-presentation. *Psychological Bulletin, 111,* 203-243.

Dickson, D. A., Hargie, O., & Morrow, N. C. (1989). *Communication skills training for health professionals.* London. Chapman and Hall.

Dubrin, A. J. (2000). *Applying psychology & individual organizational effectiveness.* (5th ed.). Upper Saddle River, NJ: Prentice Hall.

Edwards, B. (1999). *The new drawing on the right side of the brain.* New York: Jeremy P. Tarcher/Putnam.

Friedman, M., & Rosenman, R. H. (1974). *Type A behavior and your heart.* New York: Knopf.

Fujishin, R. (2000). *Creating communication: Exploring and expanding your fundamental communication skills.* San Francisco: Acada Books.

Goleman, D. (2001). Emotional intelligence: Issues in paradigm building. In C. Cherniss & D. Goleman (Eds.), *The emotionally intelligent workplace* (pp. 13-26). San Francisco: Jossey Bass.

Hall, E. T. (1990). *The hidden dimension.* New York: Anchor Books.

Harter, S. (1999). *The construction of the self: A developmental perspective.* New York: Guilford.

Katz, S. (1988, October). *Untitled presentation.* Paper presented at the Mid-Atlantic Beauty Conference.

Long, V. O. (1996). *Communication skills in helping relationships: A framework for facilitating personal growth.* Pacific Grove, CA: Brooks Cole.

Markus, H., & Nurius, P. (1986). Possible selves. *American Psychologist, 41,* 954-969.

Maslow, A. H. (1970). *Motivation and personality* (2nd ed.). New York: Harper & Row.

Mossholder, K. W., Bedeian, A. G., & Armenakis, A. (1982). Group process-work outcome relationships: A note of the moderating impact of self-esteem. *Academy of Management Journal, 25,* 575-585.

Plotnik, R. (2002). *Introduction to psychology* (6th ed.). Belmont, CA: Wadsworth.

Reis, H. T., Wilson, I., Monestere, C., Bernstein, S., Clark, K., Seidl, E., et al. (1990). What is smiling is beautiful and good. *European Journal of Social Psychology, 20,* 259-267.

Robbins, A. (1986). *Unlimited power.* New York: Ballantine.

Salovey, P., & Mayer, J. D. (1990). Emotional intelligence. *Imagination, Cognition, and Personality, 9,* 185-211.

Selye, H. (1952). *The story of the adaptation syndrome.* Montreal: Acta.

Seta, C. E., Paulus, P. B., & Baron, R. A. (2000). *Effective human relations: A guide to people at work.* Needham Heights, MA: Allyn & Bacon.

Sperry, R. W. (1982). Some effects of disconnecting the cerebral hemispheres. *Science, 217,* 1223-1226, 1250.

Springer, S. P., & Deutsch, G. (1998). *Left brain, right brain.* New York: W. H. Freeman.

Troc, K. (2003). *Success in sales and marketing.* Unpublished manuscript.

Weiten, W. (2002). *Psychology: Themes and variations* (5th ed.). Pacific Grove, CA: Thomson Learning.

Zimbardo, P. G. (1977). *Shyness: What it is and what you can do about it.* Reading, MA: Addison-Wesley.

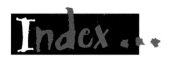

Index . . .

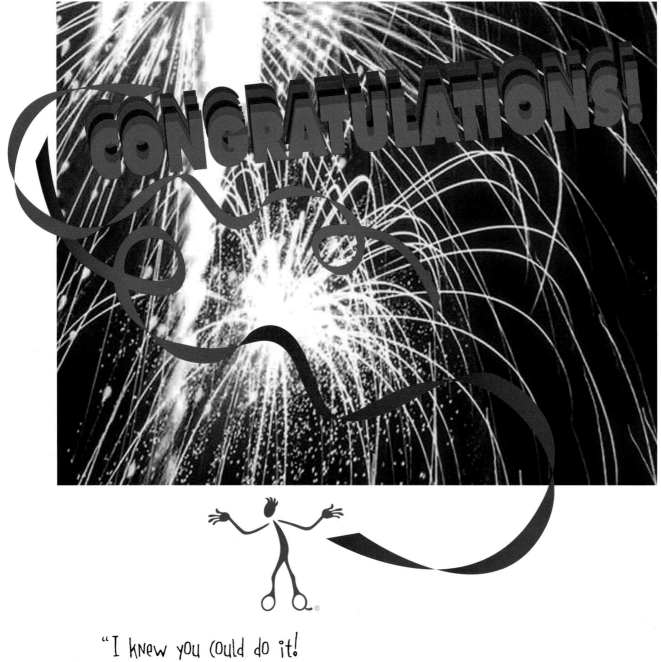

"I knew you could do it!
The new knowledge you have acquired is just the beginning.
Through continuous investigation and experimentation, you'll
be able to achieve all of your goals!"

CLiC Classmates Sign In ...

School _____   Class of _____

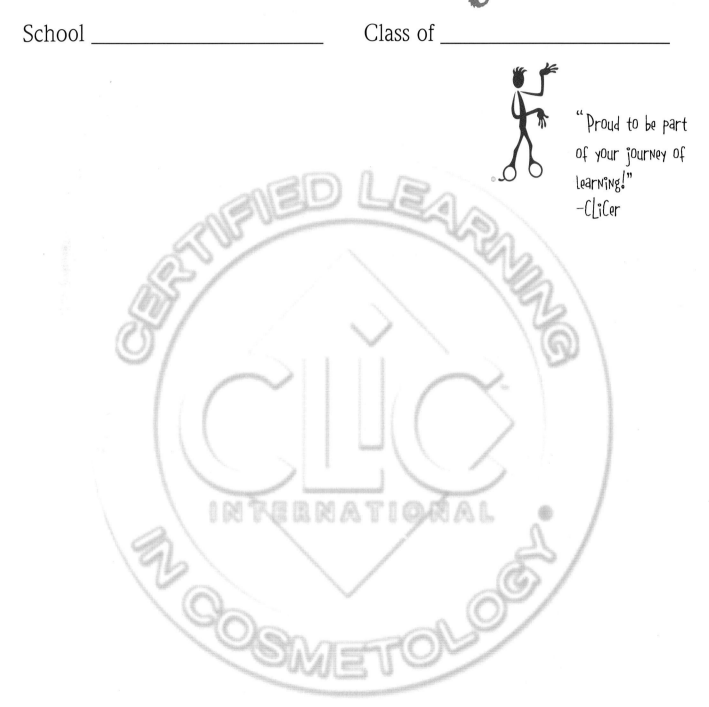

"Proud to be part of your journey of learning!"
—CLiCer

Thank you for joining our professional team of great stylists!

 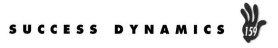

CONGRATULATIONS!

Now that you have completed your journey through the **Success Dynamics** module, you are ready to take the Student Certification Exam. With a passing grade, you will receive official certification documenting that you have mastered the skills presented in the **Success Dynamics** module.

As you continue on your journey through each of the **CLiC** learning modules, you will receive a certificate for each module completed successfully. After completing all modules with passing grades, you will receive a **CLiC** masters certification award.

Best of success to you!

For more information call:
CLiC INTERNATIONAL®
1.800.207.5400
info@clicusa.com

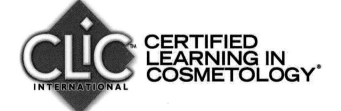

"Way to go! I knew you could do it!"

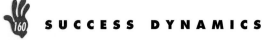